Fastest Anti-Inflammatory Diet Collections

Fit and Healthy Breakfast Recipes for Busy People

Zac Gibson

© **Copyright 2021 - All rights reserved.**

The content contained within this book may not be reproduced, duplicated or transmitted without direct written permission from the author or the publisher.

Under no circumstances will any blame or legal responsibility be held against the publisher, or author, for any damages, reparation, or monetary loss due to the information contained within this book. Either directly or indirectly.

Legal Notice:

This book is copyright protected. This book is only for personal use. You cannot amend, distribute, sell, use, quote or paraphrase any part, or the content within this book, without the consent of the author or publisher.

Disclaimer Notice:

Please note the information contained within this document is for educational and entertainment purposes only. All effort has been executed to present accurate, up to date, and reliable, complete information. No warranties of any kind are declared or implied. Readers acknowledge that the author is not engaging in the rendering of legal, financial, medical or professional advice. The content within this book has been derived from various sources. Please consult a licensed professional before attempting any techniques outlined in this book.

By reading this document, the reader agrees that under no circumstances is the author responsible for any losses, direct or indirect, which are incurred as a result of the use of information contained within this document, including, but not limited to, — errors, omissions, or inaccuracies.

Table of Contents

Watermelon Salad 8

Peppers and Olives Salad 10

Sweet Potato, Spinach, and Eggs Mix 12

Avocado and Mango Salad......................................14

Brussels Sprouts Eggs with Turmeric 16

Strawberries and Spinach Bowls 18

Collard and Spinach Oatmeal.................................20

Spinach, Kale and Quinoa Salad............................22

Fennel, Kale and Barley Salad 24

Chili Carrot and Sweet Potato Mix 26

Jalapeno Cucumber Bowls......................................28

Zucchinis, Arugula, and Barley Mix 30

Avocado and Pepper Eggs Mix 32

Olives Frittata with Shallots...................................34

Berries Coconut Mix 36

Cucumber, Spinach, and Olives Salad...................38

Sweet Potato Bowls...40

Shallots Cucumber Omelet 42

Cinnamon Oatmeal with Maple Syrup 44

Chili Broccoli Salad 46

Spinach, Kale, and Olives Bowls 48

Cherry Tomato and Orange Salad 50

Pear and Kale Salad 52

Berries and Cantaloupe Salad 54

Cauliflower and Eggs Mix 56

Cranberries Nuts Oats 58

Avocado and Banana Smoothie 60

Beet Tomato Salad 62

Quinoa with Strawberries and Maple Syrup 64

Carrots and Quinoa Mix 66

Avocado and Tomatoes Salad 68

Black Beans, Scallions, and Eggs Mix 70

Avocado, Pepper and Corn Salad 72

Cherry Tomatoes and Eggs 74

Zucchini Onion Spread 76

Watermelon, Arugula and Quinoa Salad 78

Portuguese Salad 80

Tomato Eggs 82

Vanilla Pears 84

Strawberry Salad 86

Spinach Frittata 88

Granola Bars 90

Kale Salad.. 92

Quinoa Salad... 94

Shredded Carrot Bowl... 96

Italian Style Salad... 98

Sprouts Salad.. 100

Corn Bowl 102

Lemon Tomatoes 104

Avocado Salad... 106

Watermelon Salad

Prep Time:
10 minutes
Cook Time:
0 minutes
Serve: 2

Ingredients:

- ½ teaspoon agave nectar
- 2 tablespoons lemon juice
- 1 tablespoon extra-virgin olive oil
- 1 jalapeno, seeded and chopped
- 12 ounces watermelon, chopped
- 1 red onion, thinly sliced
- ½ cup chopped basil leaves
- 2 cups baby arugula

Directions:

1. In a bowl, toss together the watermelon with the jalapeno, onion, basil, arugula, oil, agave nectar, lemon juice, and oil.

Nutrition: calories 128, fat 8, fiber 2, carbs 16, protein 2

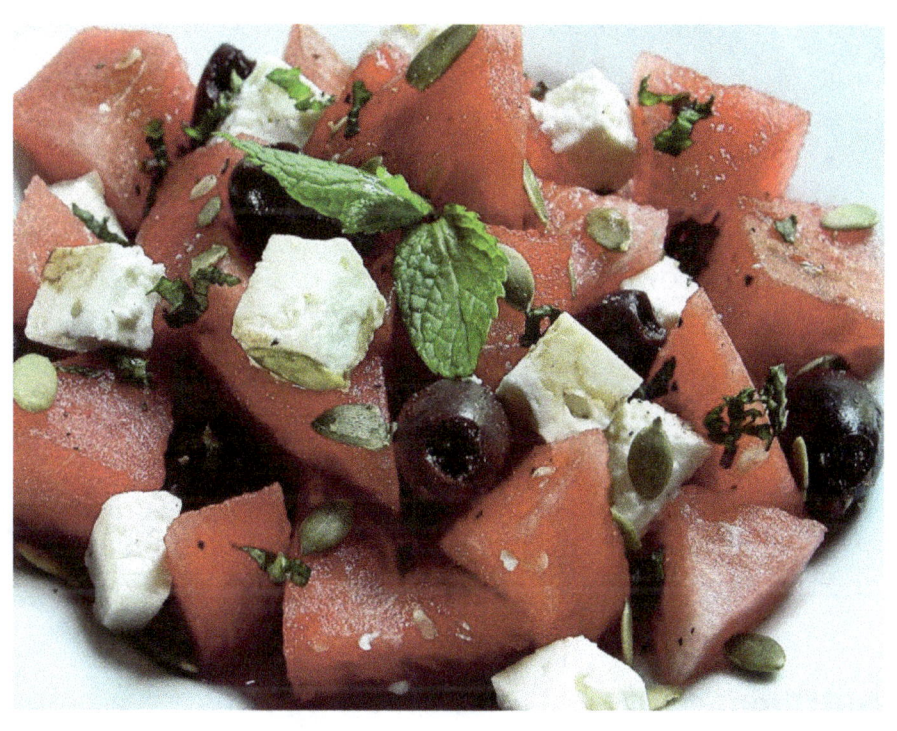

Peppers and Olives Salad

Prep Time:
10 minutes
Cook Time:
0 minutes
Serve: 4

Ingredients:

- 1 red bell pepper, cut into strips
- 1 green bell pepper, cut into strips
- 2 spring onions, chopped
- 1 cup black olives, pitted and halved
- 1 cup kalamata olives, pitted and halved A pinch of garlic powder
- A pinch of salt and black pepper
- 1 tablespoon avocado oil

Directions:

1.In a bowl, combine the bell peppers with the onions and the other ingredients, toss, divide between plates, and serve breakfast.

Nutrition: calories 221, fat 6, fiber 6, carbs 14, protein 11

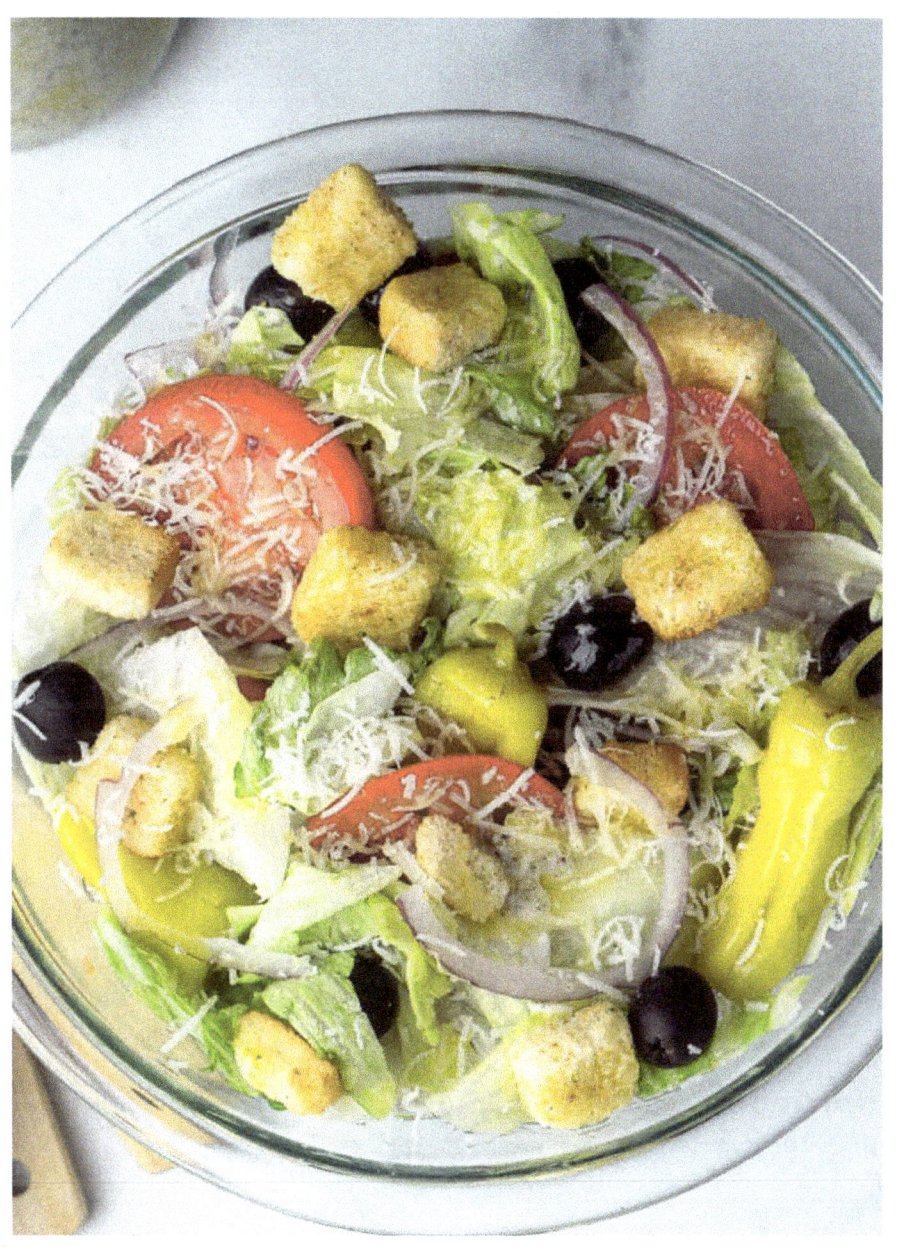

Sweet Potato, Spinach, and Eggs Mix

Prep Time:
5 minutes
Cook Time:
15 minutes
Serve: 4

Ingredients:

- A pinch of salt and black pepper
- 8 eggs, whisked
- 1 tablespoon olive oil
- 1 small yellow onion, chopped
- 2 garlic cloves, minced
- 1 cup sweet potato, peeled, and cup bed
- 1 cup baby spinach
- 1 tablespoon chives, chopped

Directions:

1. Heat a pan with the oil over medium-high heat, add the onion and the garlic and sauté for 2 minutes.

2. Add the potato, stir and cook for 3 minutes more.

3. Add the eggs and the other ingredients, cook for 10 minutes, stirring from time to time, divide between plates, and serve breakfast.

Nutrition: calories 213.3, fat 12.3, fiber 7, carbs 14, protein 2.3

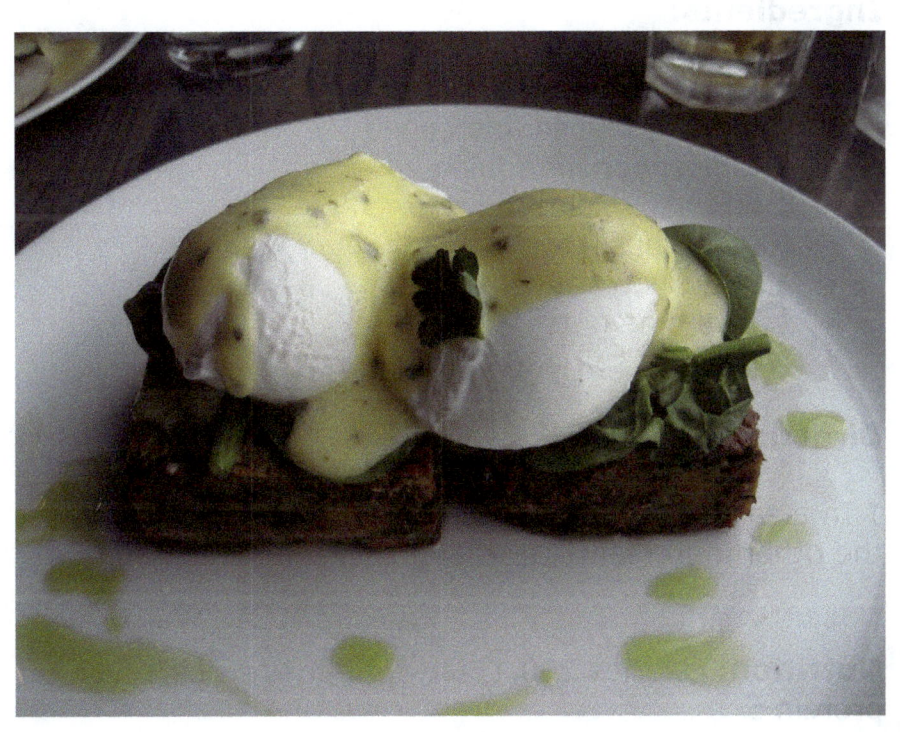

Avocado and Mango Salad

Prep Time:
5 minutes
Cook Time:
0 minutes
Serve: 2

Ingredients:

- 2 avocados, peeled, pitted, and roughly cubed
- 1 mango, peeled and cubed
- 1 tablespoon lime juice
- 1 cup baby spinach
- Handful basil, torn
- 1 tablespoon olive oil
- ¼ cup pine nuts, toasted
- A pinch of salt and black pepper

Directions:

1. In a salad bowl, mix avocados with the mango and the other ingredients, toss and serve for breakfast.

Nutrition: calories 200.1, fat 4, fiber 4, carbs 14.1, protein 5

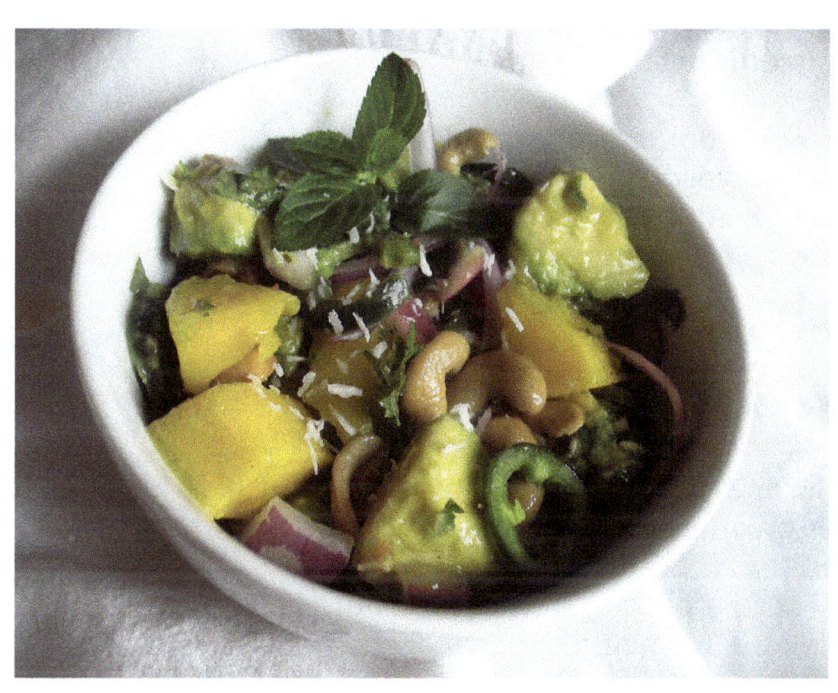

Brussels Sprouts Eggs with Turmeric

Prep Time:
10 minutes
Cook Time:
15 minutes
Serve: 4

Ingredients:

- 1 cup Brussels sprouts, shredded
- 1 yellow onion, chopped
- 8 eggs, whisked
- 1 tablespoon olive oil
- 1 tablespoon turmeric powder
- 1 tablespoon cilantro, chopped
- 1 teaspoon cumin, ground
- A pinch of salt and black pepper

1. Heat a pan with the oil over medium-high heat, add the onion and the sprouts and sauté for 5 minutes.

2. Add the eggs and the other ingredients, toss well, cook for 10 minutes more, divide between plates and serve.

Nutrition: calories 177, fat 2, fiber 6, carbs 15, protein 6

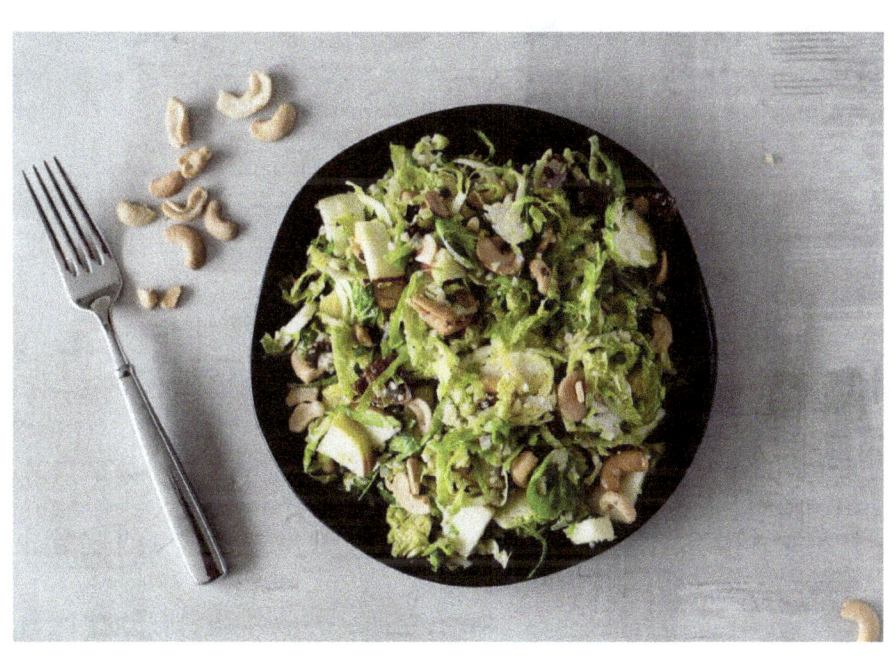

Strawberries and Spinach Bowls

Prep Time:
5 minutes
Cook Time:
0 minutes
Serve: 4

Ingredients:

- 2 cups baby spinach
- 10 strawberries, halved
- 1 tablespoon pine nuts
- 1 tablespoon almonds, chopped
- 1 tablespoon lime juice
- 1 tablespoon avocado oil

Directions:

1. In a bowl, combine the spinach with the strawberries and the other ingredients, toss and serve for breakfast.

Nutrition: calories 171, fat 3, fiber 6, carbs 15, protein 5

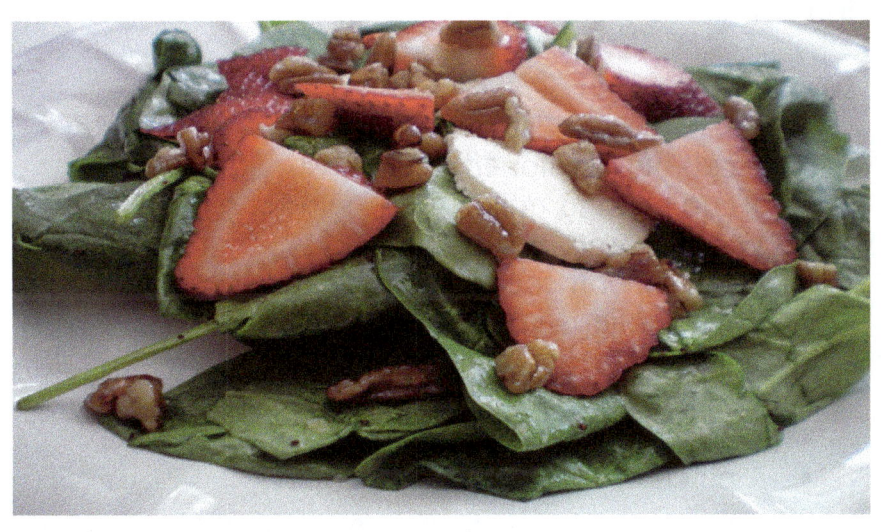

Collard and Spinach Oatmeal

Prep Time:
10 minutes
Cook Time:
20 minutes
Serve: 4

Ingredients:

- 1 cup old-fashioned oats
- 1 cup almond milk
- ½ cup water
- 1 tablespoon coconut oil, melted
- ½ cup collard greens, chopped
- ½ cup baby spinach, chopped
- A handful basil, chopped
- ½ tablespoon rosemary, chopped
- A pinch of salt and black pepper

Directions:

1. Heat a pot with the milk and the water over medium heat, add the oats, the oil, and the other ingredients, cook for 20 minutes, stirring often, divide into bowls and serve warm.

Nutrition: calories 246, fat 19.3, fiber 3.8, carbs 17.6, protein 4.1

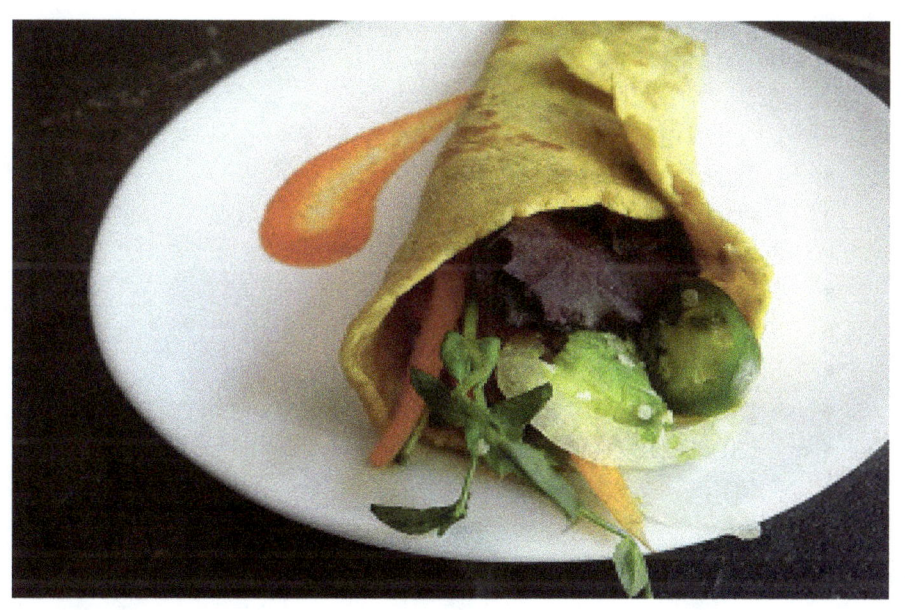

Spinach, Kale and Quinoa Salad

Prep Time:
10 minutes
Cook Time:
0 minutes
Serve: 4

Ingredients:

- 1 cup baby spinach
- 1 cup baby kale
- 2 spring onions, chopped
- 2 tablespoons olive oil
- 1 cup quinoa, cooked
- 1 carrot, shredded
- 1 red bell pepper, cut into strips
- A pinch of salt and black pepper
- 1 tablespoon lime juice
- 4 eggs, hard boiled, peeled and roughly cubed

Directions:

1. In a salad bowl, combine the quinoa with the spinach, kale and the other ingredients, toss and serve for breakfast.

Nutrition: calories 308, fat 14.1, fiber 4.4, carbs 34, protein 12.8

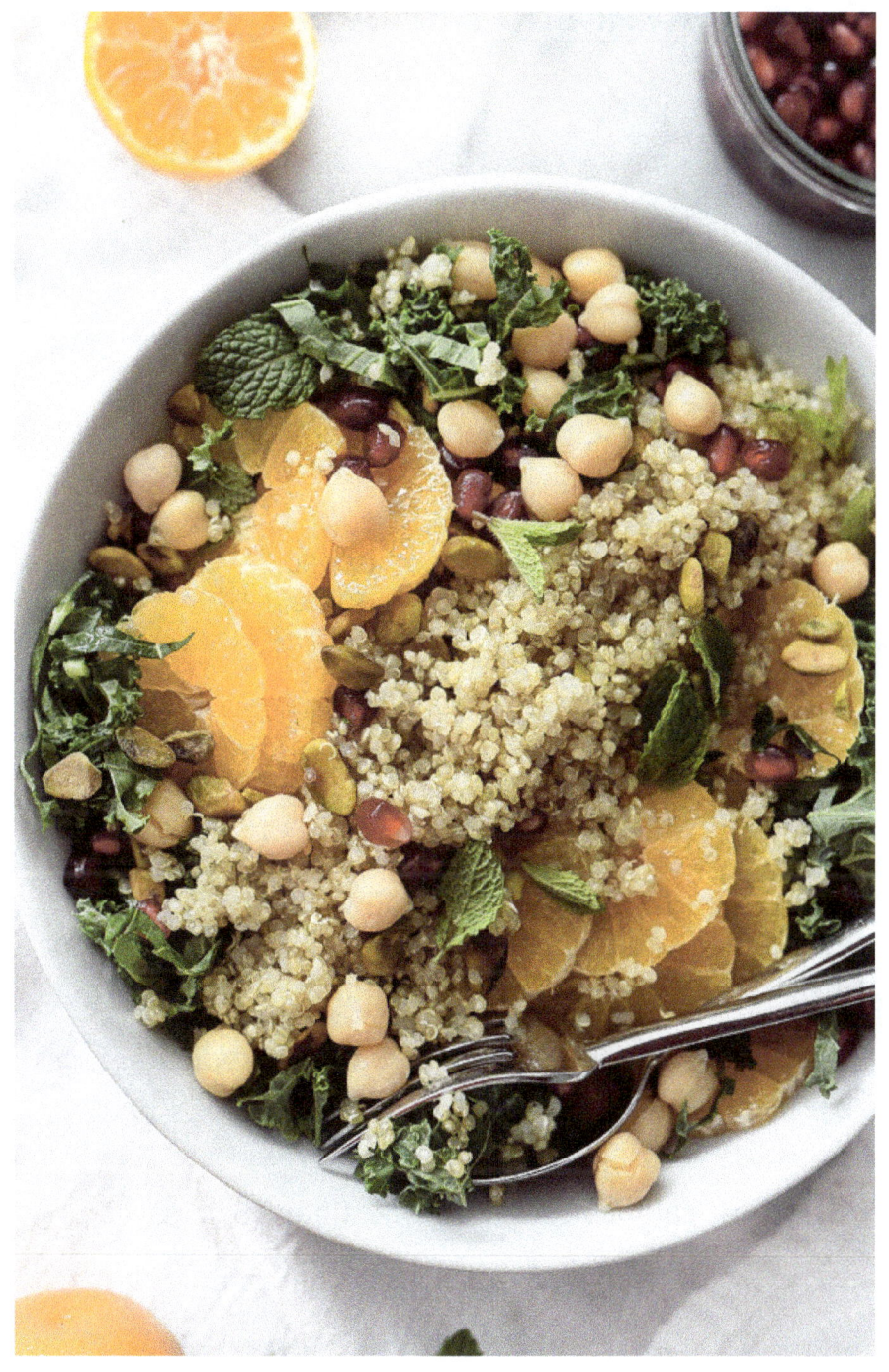

Fennel, Kale and Barley Salad

Prep Time:
10 minutes
Cook Time:
1 hour
Serve: 2

Ingredients:

- 1 cup black barley
- 3 cups water
- 2 fennel bulbs, shaved
- 1 cup baby kale
- 1 small red onion, sliced
- 2 tablespoons almonds, chopped
- 1 avocado, peeled, pitted, and cubed
- 2 tablespoons oil
- 1 tablespoon pine nuts
- 2 tablespoons balsamic vinegar
- A pinch of salt and black pepper

Directions:

1. Put the barley in a pot, add the water, salt, and pepper, bring to a simmer over medium heat, cook for 1 hour, drain, cool and transfer to a salad bowl.

2. Add the fennel, kale, and the other ingredients, toss, divide into smaller bowls, and serve for breakfast.

Nutrition: calories 545, fat 41.2, fiber 18.1, carbs 42.7, protein 9.8

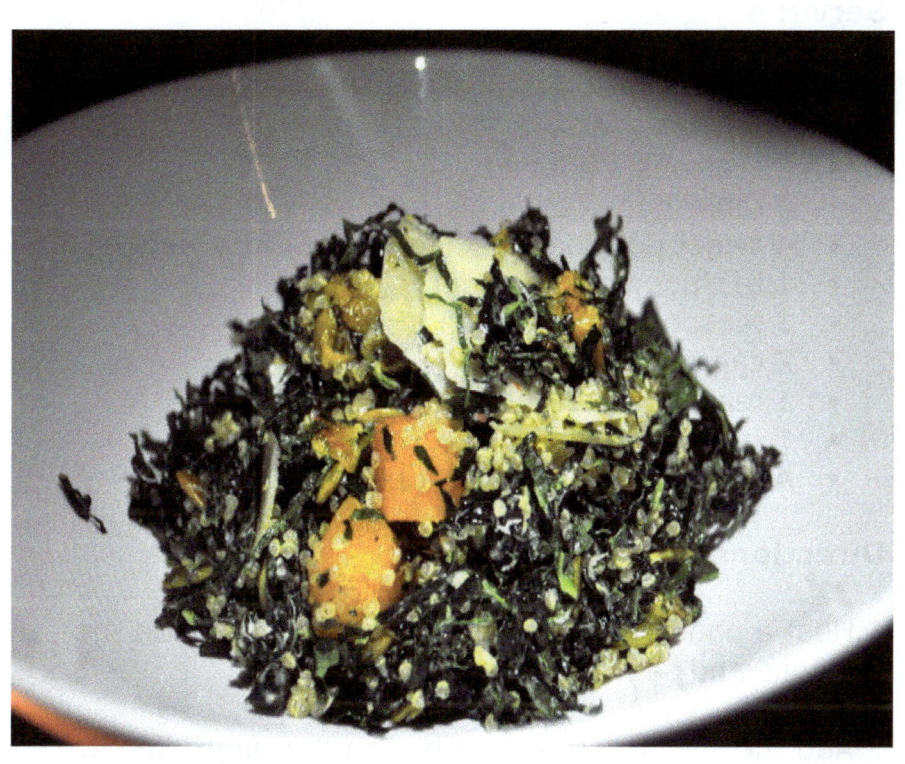

Chili Carrot and Sweet Potato Mix

Prep Time:
5 minutes
Cook Time:
20 minutes
Serve: 4

Ingredients:

- 2 scallions, chopped
- 2 tablespoons olive oil
- 4 sweet potatoes, peeled and cut into wedges
- 1 teaspoon chili powder
- 1 teaspoon hot paprika
- 2 carrots, shredded
- 1 teaspoon sesame seeds
- 1 tablespoon lime juice
- A pinch of salt and black pepper

Directions:

1. Heat a pan with the oil over medium heat, add the scallions and sauté for 2 minutes.

2. Add the sweet potatoes and the other ingredients, toss, cook for 18 minutes more, divide into bowls and serve for breakfast.

Nutrition: calories 371, fat 12.2, fiber 6, carbs 13.1, protein 5

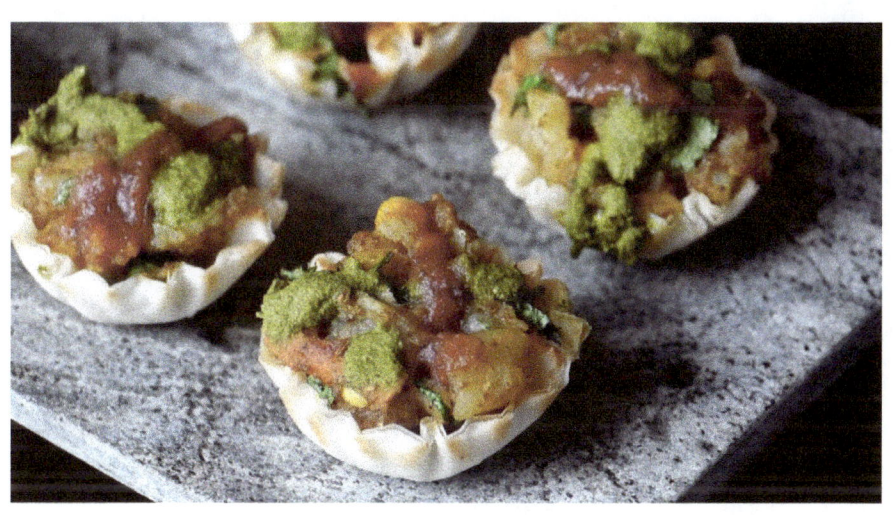

Jalapeno Cucumber Bowls

Prep Time:
5 minutes
Cook Time:
0 minutes
Serve: 4

Ingredients:

- 2 tablespoons olive oil
- 2 scallions, chopped
- 1 tablespoon lime juice
- 1 tablespoon dill, chopped
- 3 cucumbers, roughly cubed
- 2 tablespoons chives, chopped
- 1 jalapeno, chopped
- Handful basil, chopped
- 1 tablespoon almonds, crushed
- 1 tablespoon walnuts, chopped
- A pinch of salt and black pepper

Directions:

1. In a salad bowl, combine the cucumbers with the scallions and the other ingredients, toss, divide into smaller bowls, and serve breakfast.

Nutrition: calories 199, fat 4, fiber 8, carbs 15, protein 4

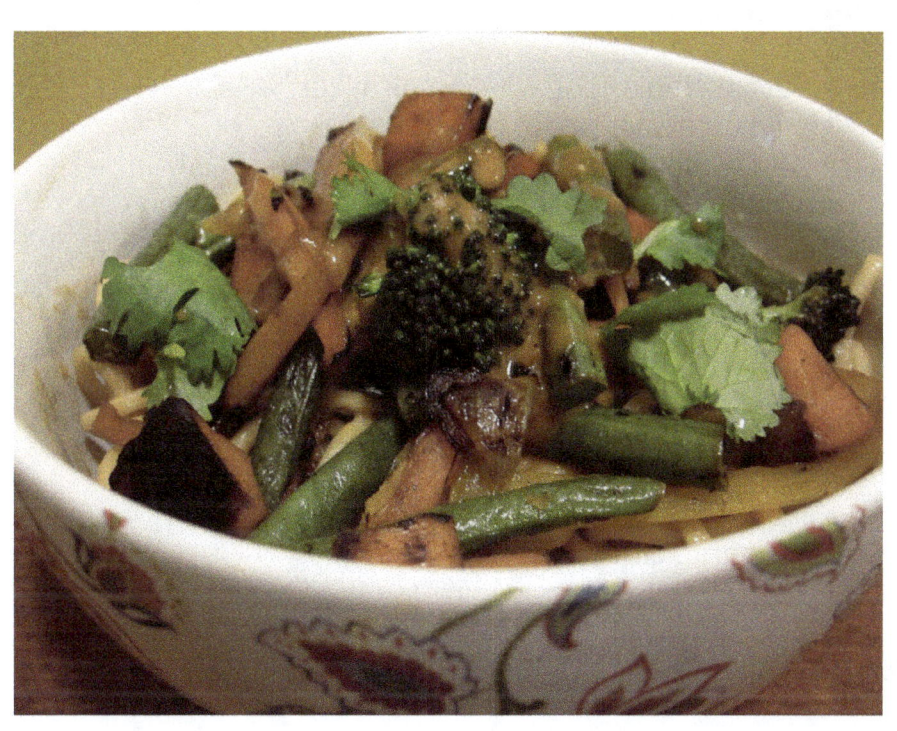

Zucchinis, Arugula, and Barley Mix

Prep Time:
10 minutes
Cook Time:
0 minutes
Serve: 4

Ingredients:

- 2 zucchinis, cut with a spiralizer
- 1 cup barley, cooked
- 2 scallions, chopped
- 1 tablespoon olive oil
- ½ teaspoon sweet paprika
- A pinch of chili powder
- 1 tablespoon lime juice
- A pinch of salt and black pepper
- 1 tablespoon oregano, chopped
- 2 cups baby arugula
- ½ cup sesame seeds paste
- 1 tablespoon balsamic vinegar
- 1 garlic clove, minced
- ½ teaspoon cumin, ground

Directions:

1.In a large bowl, combine the zucchinis with the barley, scallions, and the other ingredients, toss, divide between plates, and serve breakfast.

Nutrition: calories 226, fat 5, fiber 7, carbs 16, protein 7

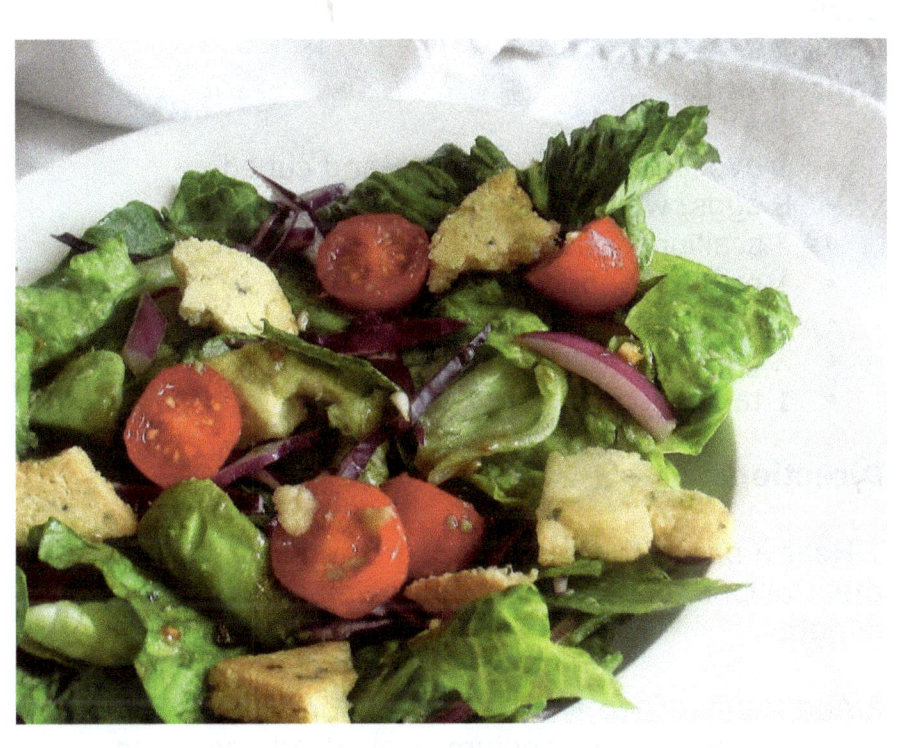

Avocado and Pepper Eggs Mix

Prep Time:
10 minutes
Cook Time:
15 minutes
Serve: 4

Ingredients:

- 1 avocado, peeled, pitted, and cubed
- 8 eggs, whisked
- 2 scallions, chopped
- 1 red bell pepper, chopped
- 2 tablespoons olive oil
- 2 garlic cloves, minced
- 1 tablespoon cilantro, chopped

Directions:

1. Heat a pan with the oil over medium-high heat, add the scallions, garlic, bell pepper, and sauté for 5 minutes.

2. Add the avocado and the other ingredients, toss, cook for 10 minutes over medium heat, divide between plates and serve.

Nutrition: calories 211, fat 2, fiber 5, carbs 16, protein 5

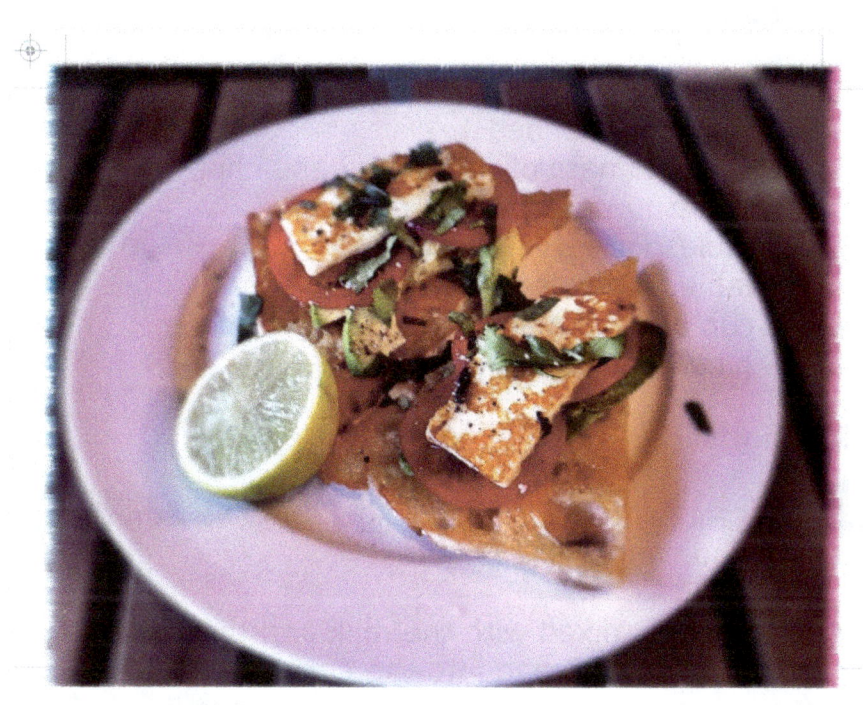

Olives Frittata with Shallots

Prep Time:
10 minutes
Cook Time:
20 minutes
Serve: 4

Ingredients:

- 8 eggs, whisked
- 2 shallots, chopped
- 1 cup kalamata olives, pitted and chopped
- 1 tablespoon coriander, chopped
- 1 tablespoon chives, chopped
- 1 tablespoon olive oil
- 1 cup almond milk
- A pinch of salt and black pepper

Directions:

1. Heat a pan with the oil over medium heat, add the shallots and sauté for 2 minutes.

2. Add the eggs mixed with the milk and the other ingredients, toss, spread into the pan, introduce the frittata in the oven and cook at 360 degrees F for 18 minutes.

3. Divide the frittata between plates and serve.

Nutrition: calories 201, fat 6, fiber 9, carbs 14, protein 6

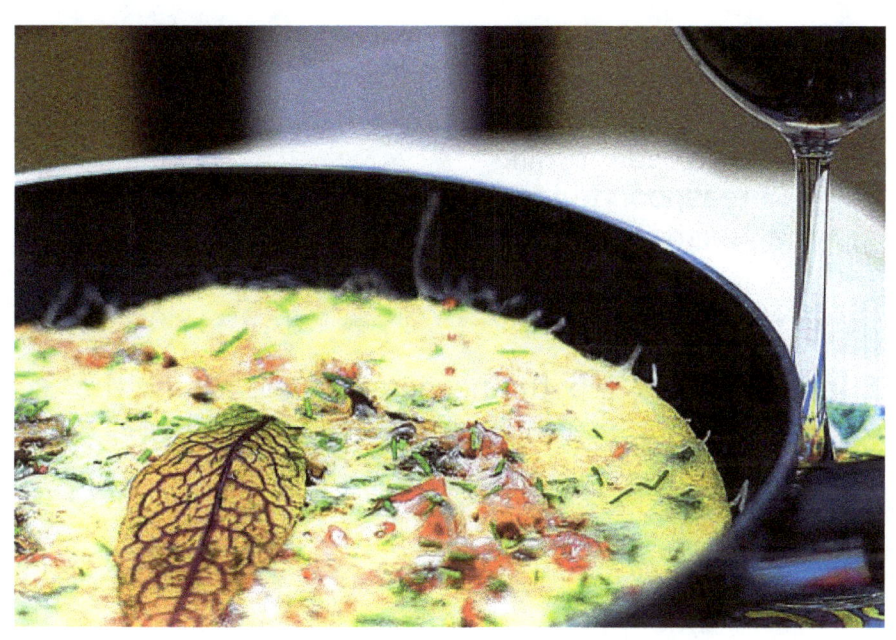

Berries Coconut Mix

Prep Time:
10 minutes
Cook Time:
15 minutes
Serve: 4

Ingredients:

- 1 cup blueberries
- 1 tablespoon coconut oil, melted
- 1/3 cup coconut flakes
- 1 cup coconut milk
- ½ teaspoon nutmeg, ground
- ½ teaspoon vanilla extract

Directions:

1.In a small pot, mix the berries with the oil and the other ingredients, toss, simmer over medium heat for 15 minutes, divide into bowls and serve.

Nutrition: calories 208, fat 2, fiber 6, carbs 16, protein 8

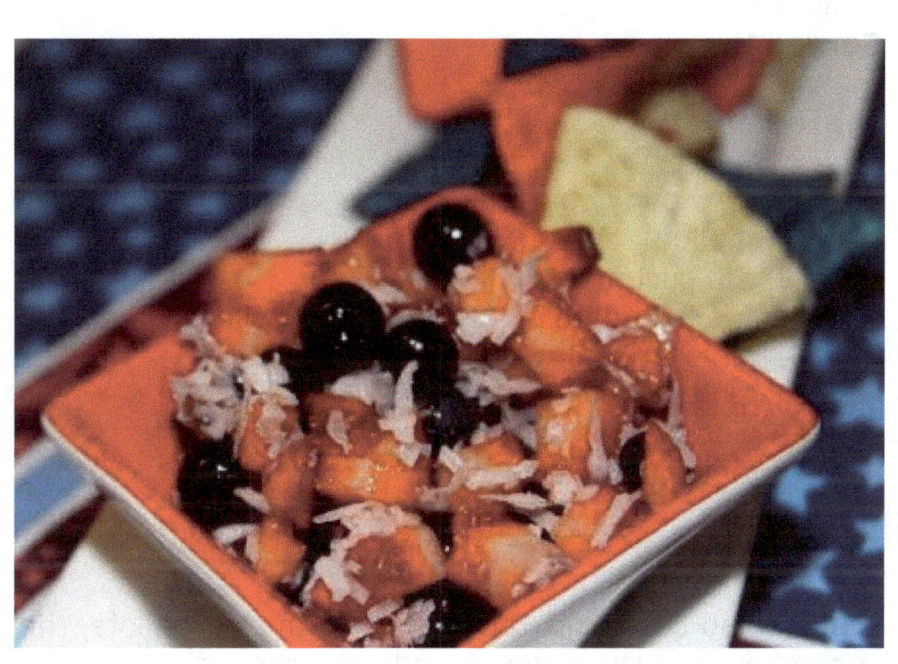

Cucumber, Spinach, and Olives Salad

Prep Time:
5 minutes
Cook Time:
0 minutes
Serve: 4

Ingredients:

- 2 cups baby spinach, torn
- 2 shallots, chopped
- 1 cup cucumber, cubed
- 1 cup kalamata olives, pitted and sliced
- 1 tablespoon chives, chopped
- 1 tablespoon balsamic vinegar
- A pinch of salt and black pepper
- 2 tablespoons olive oil

Directions:

1.In a salad bowl, mix the spinach with the shallots, the cucumber, and the other ingredients, toss, divide between plates, and serve breakfast.

Nutrition: calories 171, fat 2, fiber 5, carbs 11, protein 5

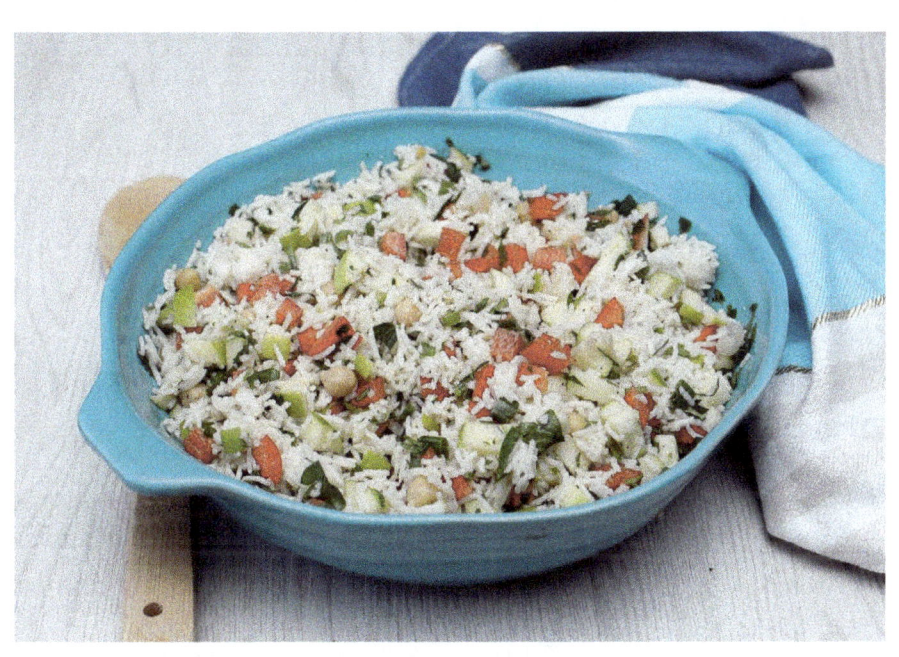

Sweet Potato Bowls

Prep Time:
5 minutes
Cook Time:
20 minutes
Serve: 4

Ingredients:

- 2 sweet potatoes, peeled and cubed
- 1 cup coconut cream
- 3 garlic cloves, minced
- 2 tablespoons olive oil
- 1 yellow onion, chopped
- 1 teaspoon cumin, ground
- 1 teaspoon turmeric powder
- 2 tablespoons parsley, chopped
- A pinch of salt and black pepper

Directions:

1. Heat a pan with the oil over medium-high heat, add the onion, garlic, cumin, turmeric, stir and sauté for 5 minutes.

2. Add the potatoes and the other ingredients, toss, cook for 15 minutes more, divide into bowls and serve for breakfast.

Nutrition: calories 188, fat 2, fiber 8, carbs 10, protein 4

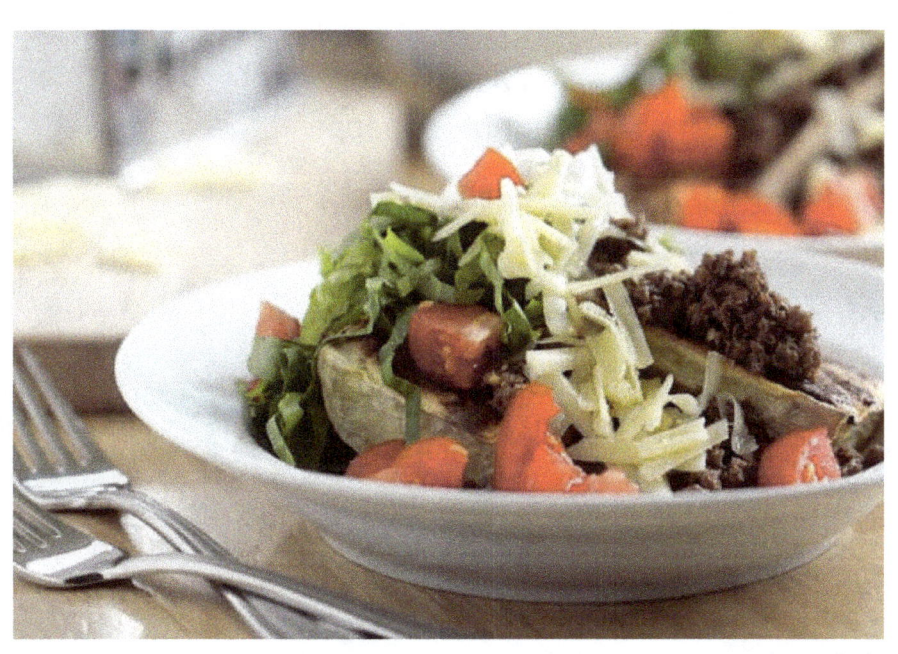

Shallots Cucumber Omelet

Prep Time:
10 minutes
Cook Time:
12 minutes
Serve: 4

Ingredients:

- 8 eggs, whisked
- 2 shallots, chopped
- A pinch of salt and black pepper
- 1 cucumber, cubed
- 1 tablespoon parsley, chopped
- 1 tablespoon olive oil

Directions:

1. Heat a pan with the oil over medium-high heat, add the shallots and sauté for 2 minutes.

2. Add the eggs mixed with the other ingredients, toss, spread into the pan, cook for 5 minutes, flip and cook for another 5 minutes.

3. Cut the omelet, divide it between plates and serve for breakfast.

Nutrition: calories 201, fat 2, fiber 5, carbs 11, protein 5

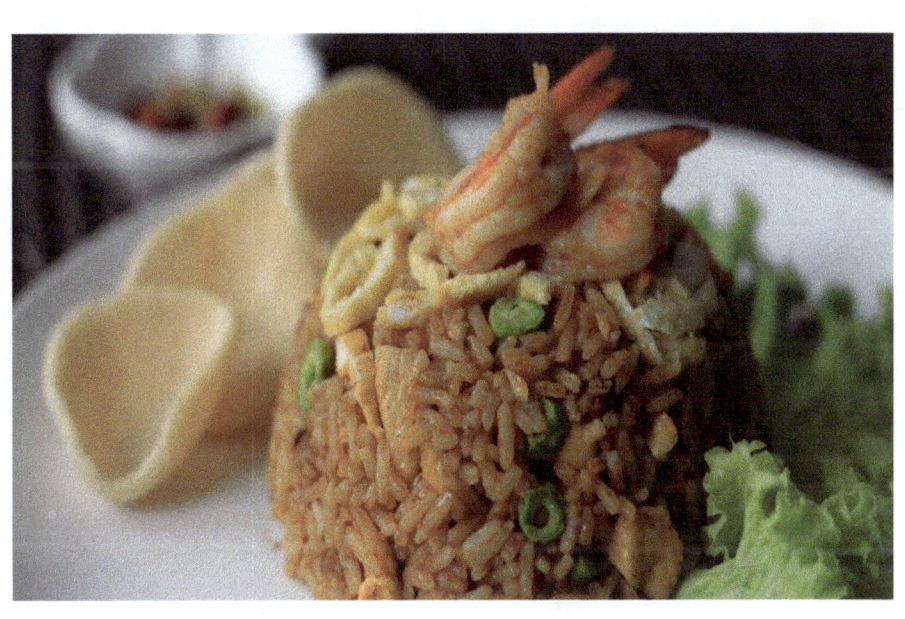

Cinnamon Oatmeal with Maple Syrup

Prep Time:
10 minutes
Cook Time:
20 minutes
Serve: 4

Ingredients:

- 2 cups coconut milk
- 1 cup old fashioned oats
- 2 tablespoons flax meal
- 1 teaspoon vanilla extract
- 2 teaspoons cinnamon powder
- 1 teaspoon maple syrup

Directions:

1.In a small pot, mix the oats with the milk and the other ingredients, toss, bring to a simmer, cook over medium heat for 20 minutes, divide into bowls and serve for breakfast.

Nutrition: calories 454, fat 32.4, fiber 7.6, carbs 35.7, protein 8.5

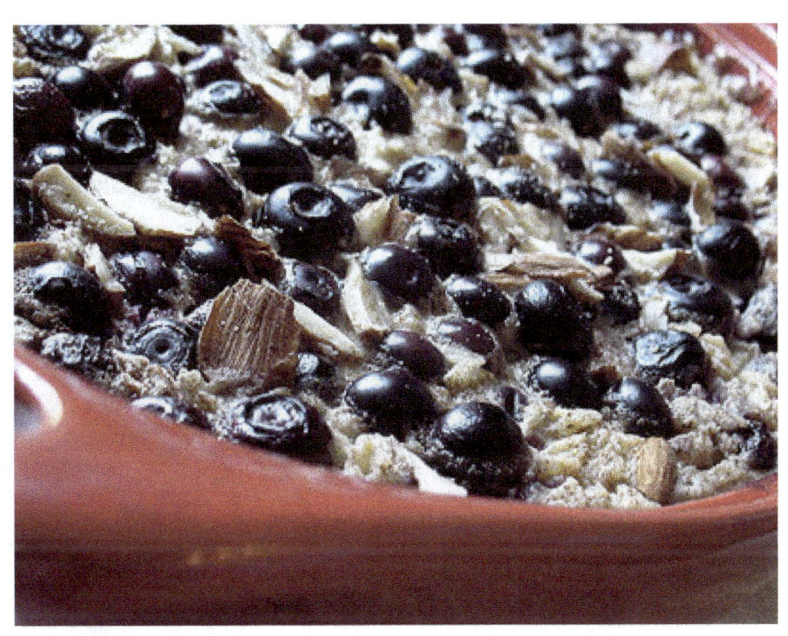

Chili Broccoli Salad

Prep Time:
10 minutes
Cook Time:
15 minutes
Serve: 4

Ingredients:

- 1 pound broccoli florets
- 1 yellow onion, chopped
- 1 tablespoon olive oil
- ½ cup coconut cream
- 1 teaspoon chili powder
- 1 teaspoon hot paprika
- 1 teaspoon garlic powder
- A pinch of salt and black pepper

Directions:

1. Heat a pan with the oil over medium-high heat, add the onion and sauté for 2 minutes.

2. Add the rest of the ingredients, toss, cook for 12 minutes over medium heat, divide into bowls, and serve breakfast.

Nutrition: calories 153, fat 11.2, fiber 4.5, carbs 12.7, protein 4.4

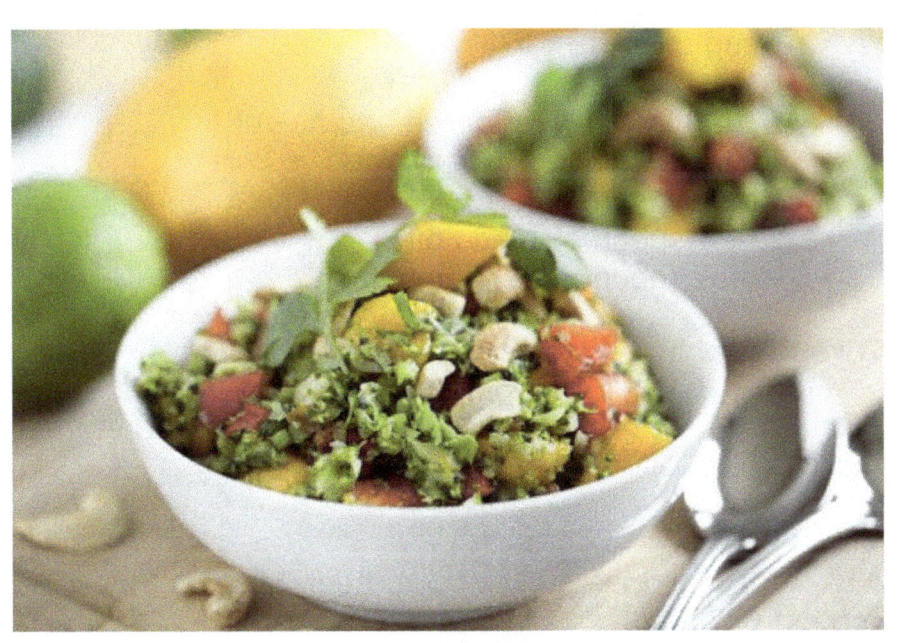

Spinach, Kale, and Olives Bowls

Prep Time:
5 minutes
Cook Time:
0 minutes
Serve: 4

Ingredients:

- 1 cup spinach, torn
- 1 cup kale, torn
- 1 cup black olives, pitted and halved
- 2 shallots, chopped
- 1 tablespoon lemon juice
- 1 tablespoon avocado oil
- 1 tablespoon mint, chopped

Directions:

1.In a bowl, mix the spinach with the kale and the other ingredients, toss, and serve breakfast.

Nutrition: calories 198, fat 6.4, fiber 2, carbs 8, protein 6

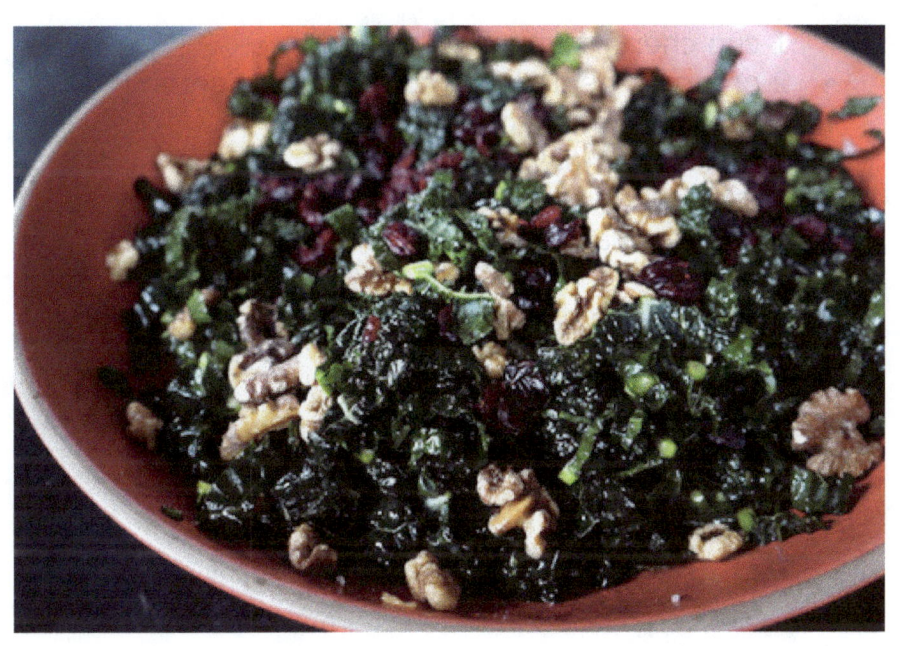

Cherry Tomato and Orange Salad

Prep Time:
6 minutes
Cook Time:
0 minutes
Serve: 4

Ingredients:

- 1 cup cherry tomatoes, halved
- 2 oranges, peeled and cut into segments
- 3 spring onions, chopped
- 1 tablespoon olive oil
- 1 tablespoon lemon juice
- A pinch of salt and black pepper
- 1 teaspoon turmeric powder

Directions:

1. In a bowl, mix the tomatoes with the oranges and the other ingredients, toss, and serve breakfast.

Nutrition: calories 255, fat 4, fiber 5, carbs 15, protein 6

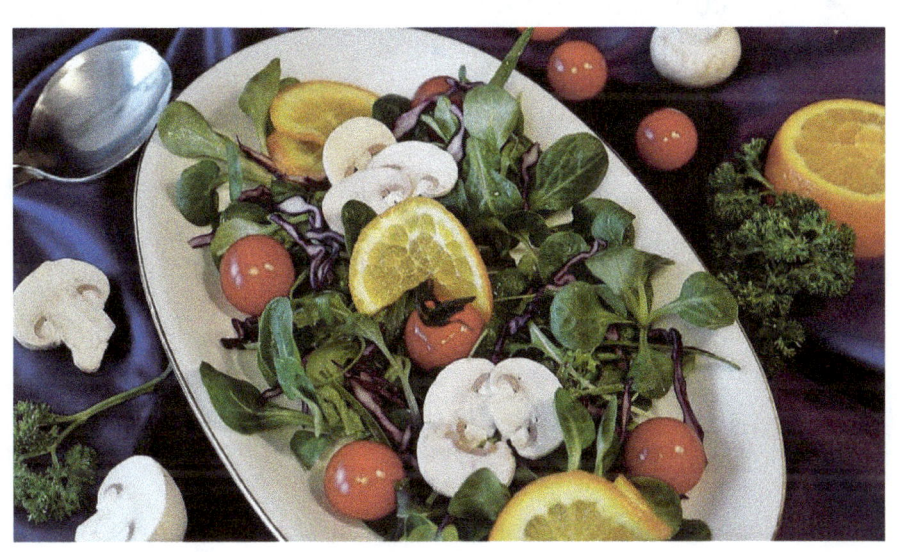

Pear and Kale Salad

Prep Time:
10 minutes
Cook Time:
15 minutes
Serve: 4

Ingredients:

- 2 cups pears, cored and cubed
- 1/3 cup coconut flakes, unsweetened
- 2 tablespoons orange juice
- 1 cup baby kale
- 1 tablespoon avocado oil

Directions:

1. In a bowl, combine the pears with the coconut and the other ingredients, toss and serve for breakfast.

Nutrition: calories 172, fat 5, fiber 7, carbs 8, protein 4

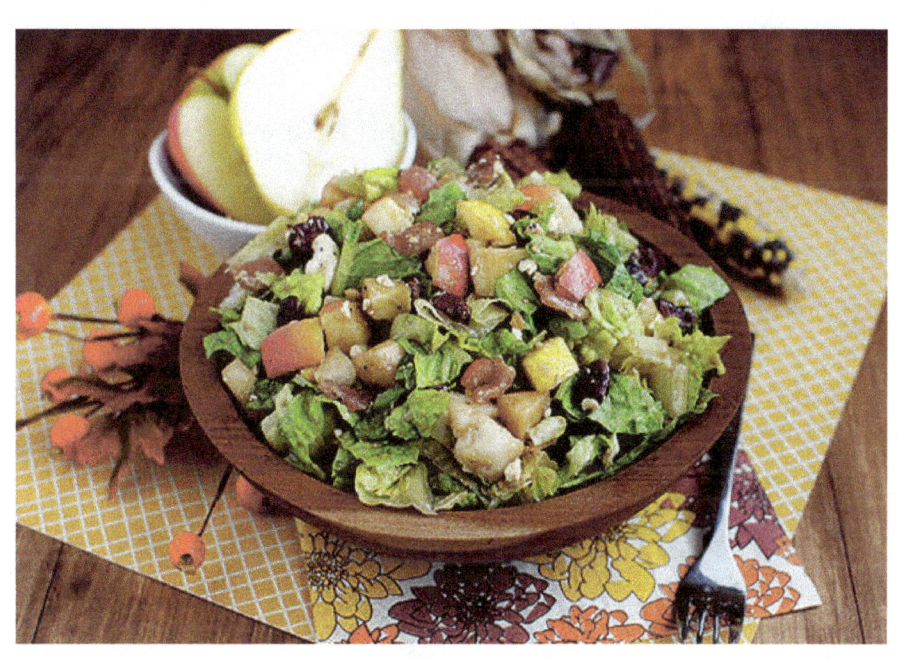

Berries and Cantaloupe Salad

Prep Time:
5 minutes
Cook Time:
0 min
Serve: 2

Ingredients:

- 2 tablespoons walnuts, chopped
- 1 cup blackberries
- 1 cup cantaloupe, peeled and cubed
- 1 tablespoon lime juice
- 1 tablespoon orange juice
- 1 teaspoon vanilla extract

Directions:

1. In a bowl, mix the blackberries with the walnuts and other ingredients, toss, divide into smaller bowls, and serve breakfast.

Nutrition: calories 90, fat 0.3, fiber 1, carbs 0, protein 5

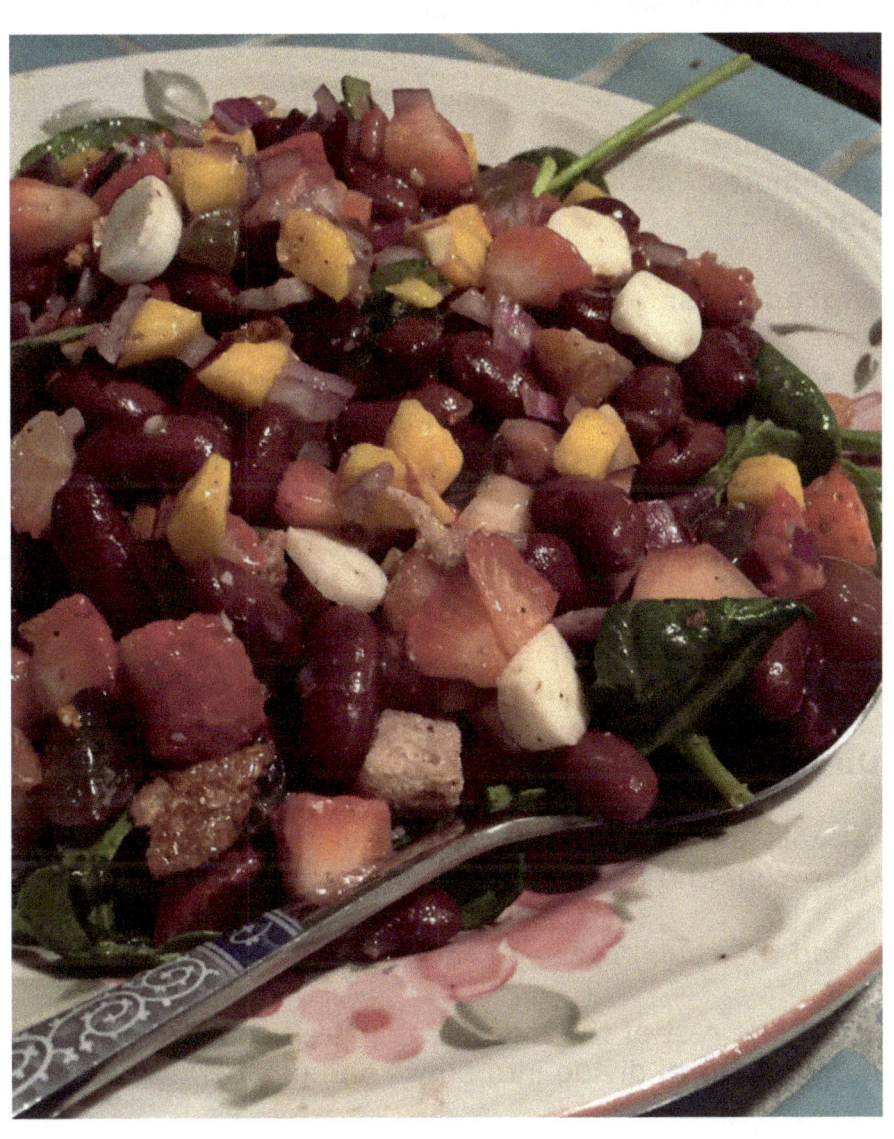

Cauliflower and Eggs Mix

Prep Time:
5 minutes
Cook Time:
20 minutes
Serve: 4

Ingredients:

- 1 cup cauliflower florets
- 1 small sweet onion, chopped
- 1 tablespoon olive oil
- 1 tablespoon lemon juice
- 1 teaspoon turmeric powder
- 1 teaspoon cumin, ground
- 2 garlic cloves, minced
- Salt and black pepper to the taste
- 4 eggs

Directions:

1. Heat a pan with the oil over medium-high heat, add the onion, and the garlic, stir and sauté for 5 minutes.

2. Add the cauliflower and cook for 5 minutes more.

3. Add the rest of the ingredients, toss, cook for 10 minutes more, divide into bowls and serve.

Nutrition: calories 214, fat 7, fiber 2, carbs 12, protein 8

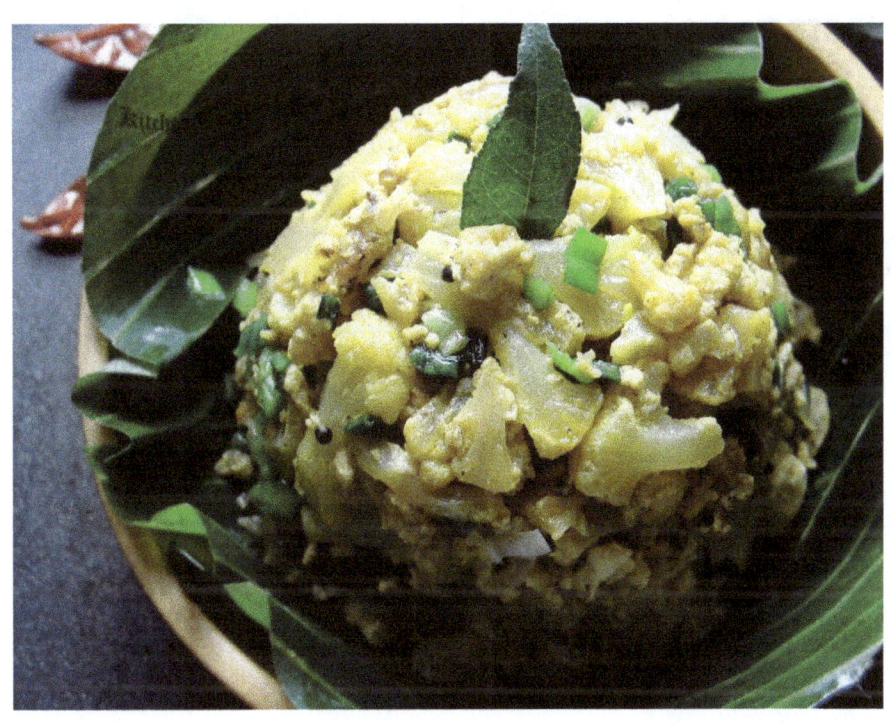

Cranberries Nuts Oats

Prep Time:
10 minutes
Cook Time:
20 minutes
Serve: 4

Ingredients

- 2 tablespoons walnuts, chopped
- 1 tablespoon almonds, chopped
- 1 cup cranberries
- 2 cups almond milk
- ½ cup old fashioned oats
- 1 teaspoon vanilla extract
- 1 teaspoon cinnamon powder

Directions:

1. In a small pot, combine the cranberries with the oats, the milk, and the other ingredients, toss, bring to a simmer and cook for 20 minutes.

2. Divide the mix into bowls and serve for breakfast.

Nutrition: calories 190, fat 1, fiber 1, carbs 7, protein 6

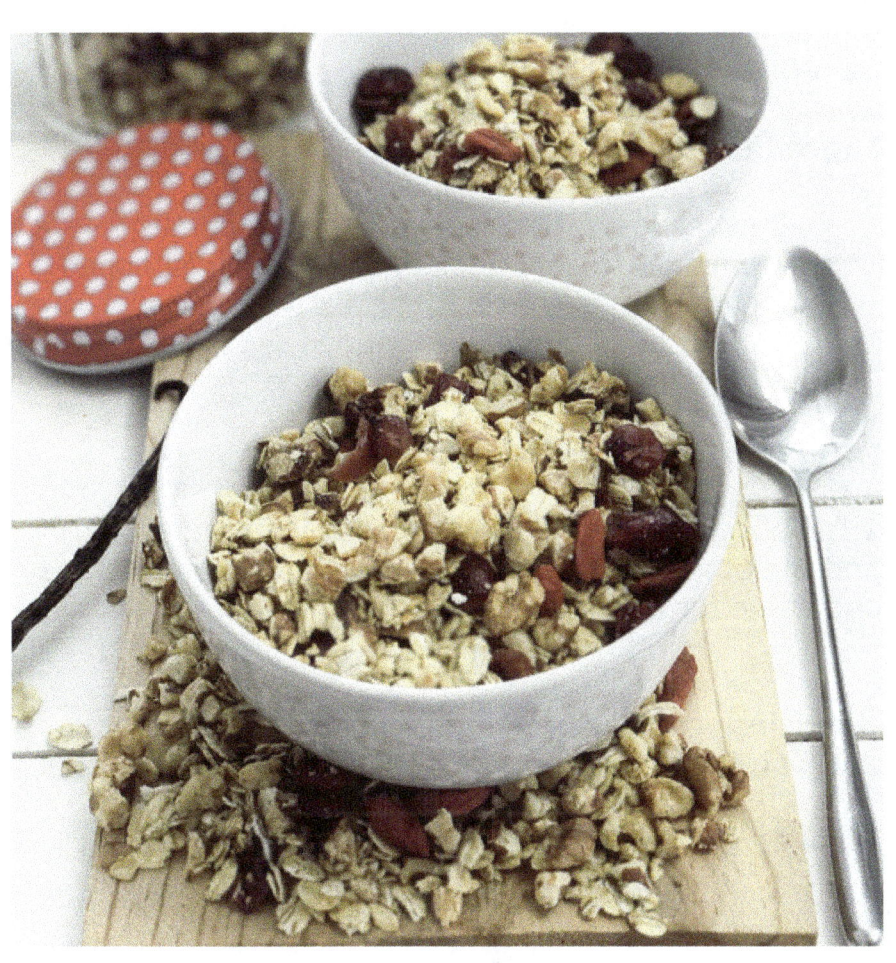

Avocado and Banana Smoothie

Prep Time:
5 minutes
Cook Time:
0 min
Serve: 4

Ingredients:

- 2 avocados, pitted, peeled, and chopped
- 1 banana, frozen, peeled, and roughly chopped
- 2 cups baby spinach
- 1 tablespoon almonds, chopped
- 2 cups almond milk, unsweetened

Directions:

1. In your blender, mix the avocados with the spinach and the other ingredients, pulse well, divide into bowls and serve for breakfast.

Nutrition: calories 519, fat 49.1, fiber 10.7, carbs 22.9, protein 5.7

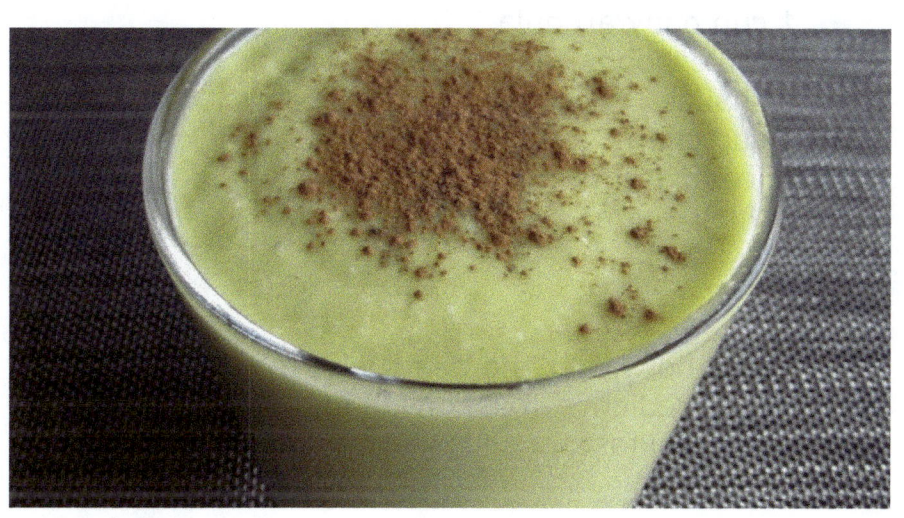

Beet Tomato Salad

Prep Time:
5 minutes
Cook Time:
0 minutes
Serve: 4

Ingredients:

- 2 cups beets, baked, peeled, and cubed
- 1 cup baby arugula
- 2 tablespoons olive oil
- 2 shallots, chopped
- 1 cup cherry tomatoes, halved
- Juice of 1 lime
- ¼ inch ginger, grated

Directions:

1. In a salad bowl, mix the beets with the arugula and the other ingredients, toss, divide into smaller bowls, and serve breakfast.

Nutrition: calories 114, fat 7.3, fiber 2.4, carbs 12/4, protein 2.2

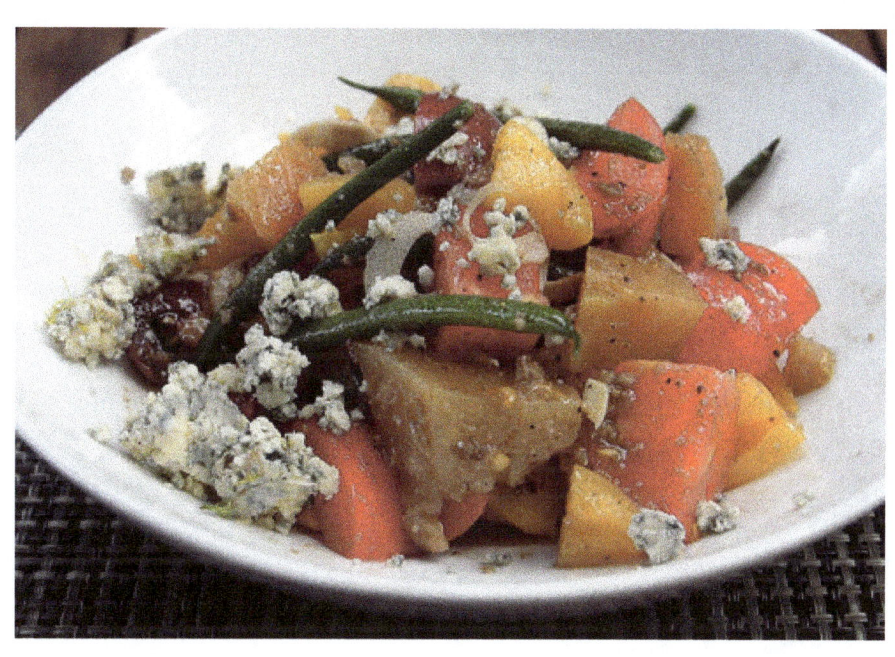

Quinoa with Strawberries and Maple Syrup

Prep Time: 5 minutes
Cook Time: 0 minutes
Serve: 4

Ingredients:

- 2 cups quinoa, cooked
- 1 cup strawberries, halved
- 1 tablespoon maple syrup
- ½ tablespoon lime juice
- 1 teaspoon vanilla extract

Directions:

1. In a bowl, mix the quinoa with the strawberries and the other ingredients, toss, divide into smaller bowls, and serve breakfast.

Nutrition: calories 170, fat 5.3, fiber 6, carbs 6.8, protein 5

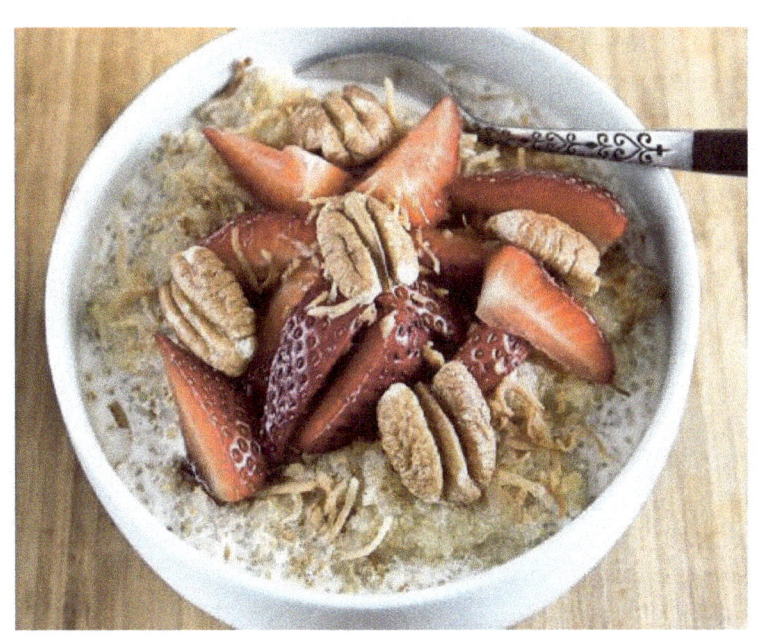

Carrots and Quinoa Mix

Prep Time:
5 minutes
Cook Time:
10 minutes
Serve: 4

Ingredients:

- 2 tablespoon maple syrup
- 1 tablespoon almonds, chopped
- 2 cups carrots, shredded
- 1 cup quinoa, cooked
- ¼ teaspoon turmeric powder
- 2 tablespoons sesame seeds
- 1 tablespoon lime juice

Directions:

1. In a salad bowl, combine the carrots with the quinoa and the other ingredients, toss, divide into ramekins, cook at 350 degrees F for 10 minutes and serve for breakfast.

Nutrition: calories 150, fat 3, fiber 2, carbs 6, protein 8

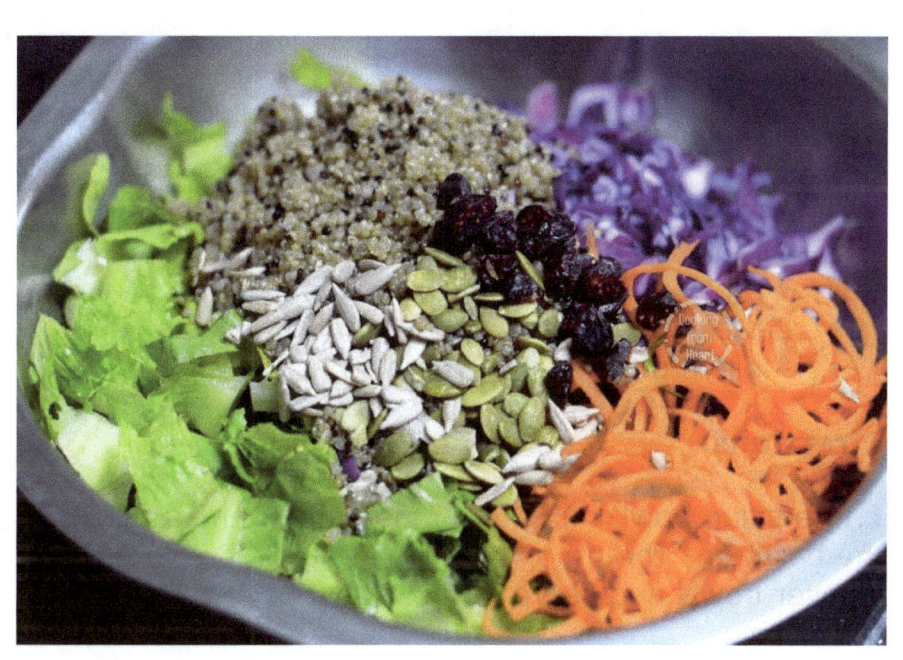

Avocado and Tomatoes Salad

Prep Time:
5 minutes
Cook Time:
0 minutes
Serve: 4

Ingredients:

- 2 cups cherry tomatoes, halved
- 2 scallions, chopped
- 1 tablespoon basil, chopped
- 1 avocado, peeled, pitted and cubed
- 2 tablespoons oregano, chopped
- 1 tablespoon mint, chopped
- 2 tablespoons balsamic vinegar
- 2 tablespoons olive oil
- A pinch of salt and black pepper

Directions:

1.In a salad bowl, mix the tomatoes with the scallions, the basil, and the other ingredients, toss, divide into smaller bowls and serve for breakfast.

Nutrition: calories 140, fat 2, fiber 3, carbs 6, protein 8

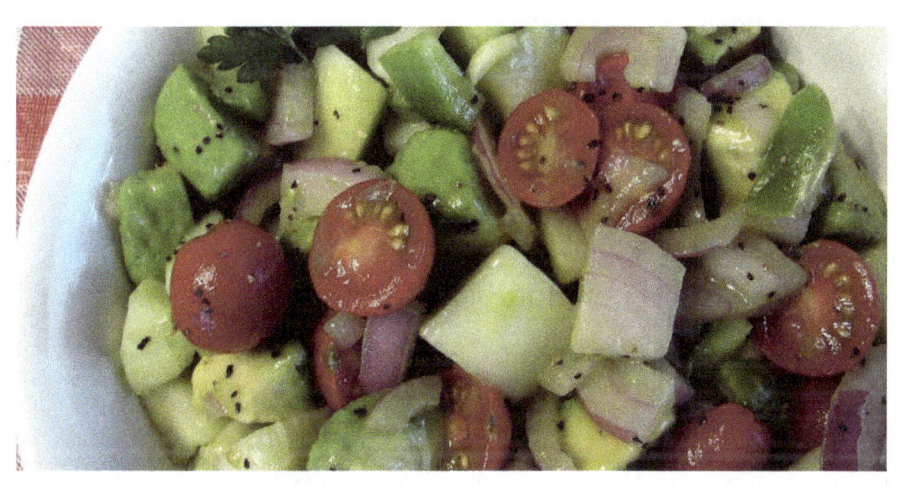

Black Beans, Scallions, and Eggs Mix

Prep Time:
5 minutes
Cook Time:
15 minutes
Serve: 4

Ingredients:

- 1 cup canned black beans, drained and rinsed
- 2 green onions, chopped
- 6 eggs, whisked
- ½ teaspoon cumin, ground
- 1 teaspoon chili powder
- 2 scallions, chopped
- 1 tablespoon olive oil
- ½ cup cilantro, chopped
- 2 tablespoons pine nuts
- A pinch of salt and black pepper

Directions:

1. Heat a pan with the oil over medium heat, add the scallions, green onions, and pine nuts, stir and cook for 2 minutes.

2. Add the beans and cook them for 3 minutes more.

3. Add the eggs and the rest of the ingredients and cook for 10 minutes more, stirring often.

4.Divide everything between plates and serve for breakfast.

Nutrition: calories 140, fat 4, fiber 2, carbs 7, protein 8

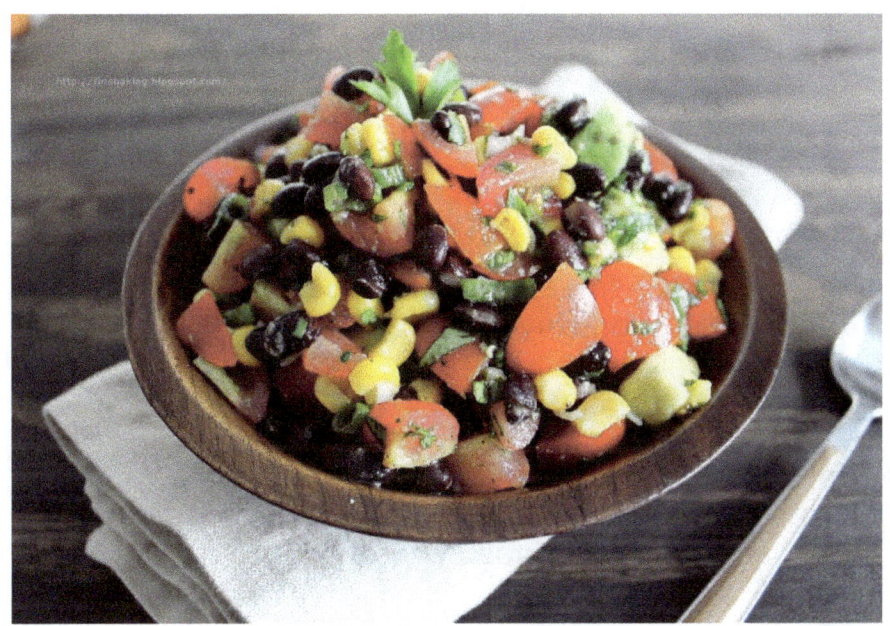

Avocado, Pepper and Corn Salad

Prep Time:
5 minutes
Cook Time:
0 minutes
Serve: 4

Ingredients:

- 2 avocados, pitted, peeled and cubed
- 1 cup corn
- 2 spring onions, chopped
- 2 red bell peppers, roughly chopped
- 2 tablespoons olive oil
- 1 tablespoon lime juice
- A pinch of salt and black pepper
- 1 tablespoon chives, chopped

Directions:

1.In a salad bowl, mix the corn with the avocado and the other ingredients, toss well, divide into smaller bowls, and serve breakfast.

Nutrition: calories 140, fat 3, fiber 2, carbs 6, protein 9

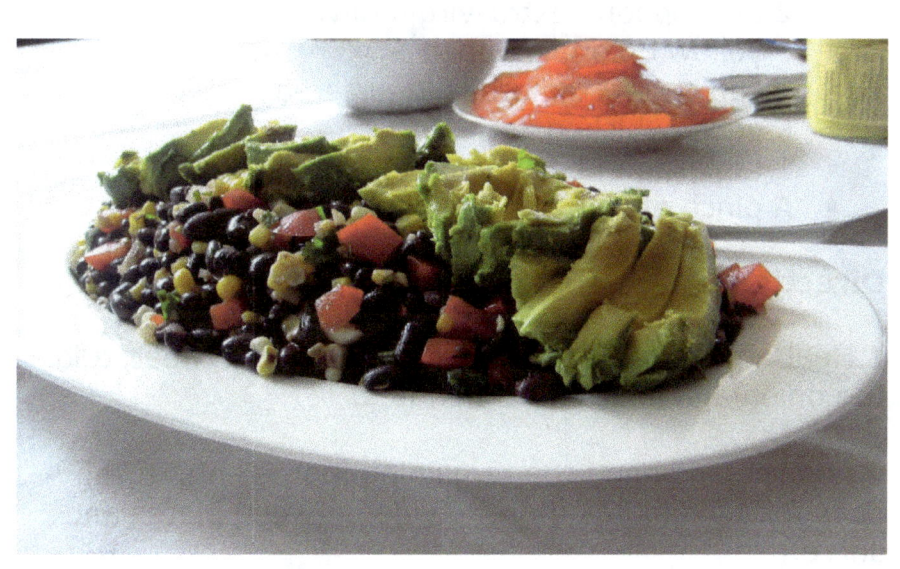

Cherry Tomatoes and Eggs

Prep Time:
5 minutes
Cook Time:
15 minutes
Serve: 4

Ingredients:

- 2 tablespoons extra-virgin olive oil
- 1 yellow onion, chopped
- 1 cup cherry tomatoes, quartered
- 6 eggs, whisked
- 1 tablespoon basil, chopped
- A pinch of salt and black pepper

Directions:

1. Heat a pan with the oil over medium-high heat, add the onion and sauté for 5 minutes.

2. Add the eggs and the remaining ingredients, toss, cook for 10 minutes more, divide between plates and serve.

Nutrition: calories 100, fat 1, fiber 2, carbs 2, protein 6

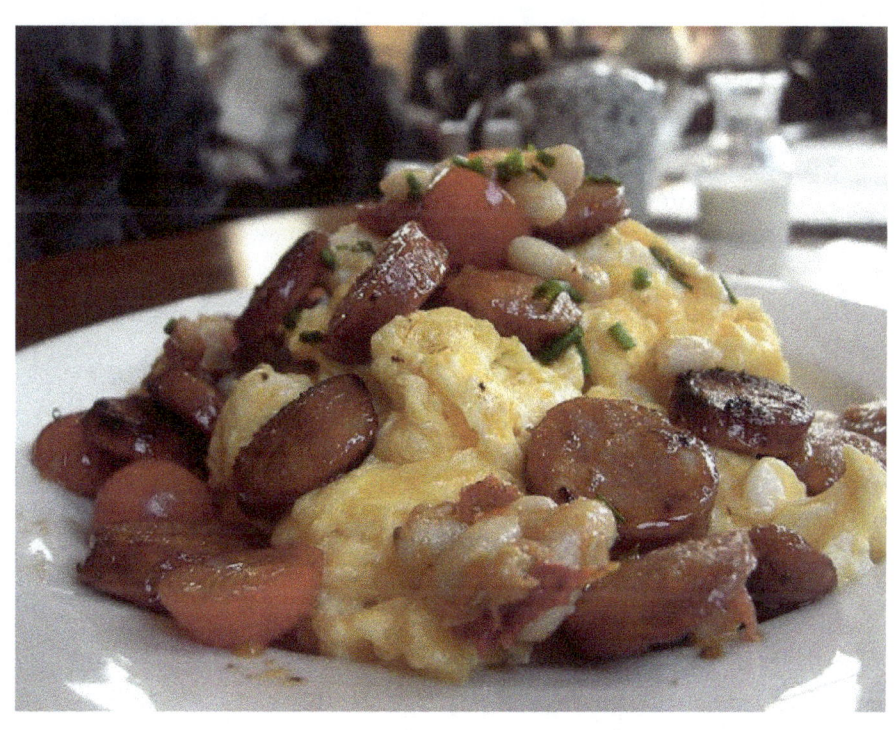

Zucchini Onion Spread

Prep Time:
10 minutes
Cook Time:
15 minutes
Serve: 4

Ingredients:

- 1 pound zucchini, chopped
- 1 yellow onion, chopped
- 1 tablespoon coconut cream
- ¼ cup veggie stock
- 2 tablespoons olive oil
- 2 tablespoons lemon juice
- ¼ cup parsley, chopped
- A pinch of salt and black pepper

Directions:

1. Heat a pan with the oil over medium heat, add the onion, stir and cook for 2 minutes.

2. Add the zucchinis and the other ingredients, stir, bring to a simmer, cook for 13 minutes more, blend using an immersion blender, divide into bowls and serve as a morning spread.

Nutrition: calories 102, fat 8.3, fiber 2.1, carbs 7.1, protein 1.9

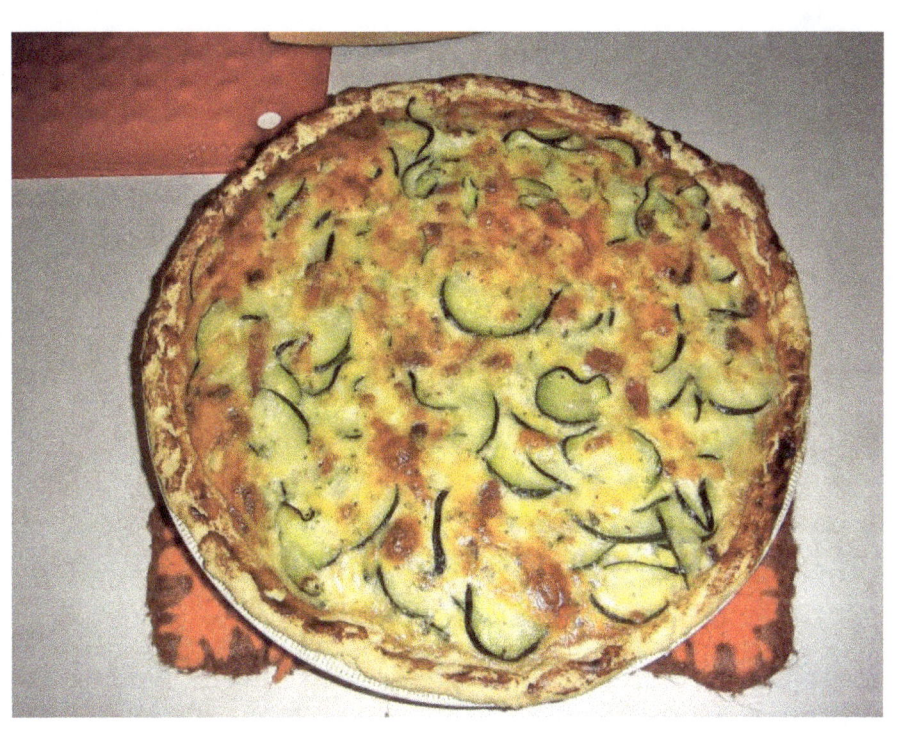

Watermelon, Arugula and Quinoa Salad

Prep Time:
10 minutes
Cook Time:
0 min
Serve: 4

Ingredients:

- ½ teaspoon maple syrup
- 2 tablespoons lemon juice
- 1 tablespoon avocado oil
- 1 cup watermelon, peeled and cubed
- 1 cup baby arugula
- 1 cup quinoa, cooked
- ½ cup basil leaves, chopped

Directions:

1. In a bowl, mix the watermelon with the arugula and the other ingredients, toss and serve for breakfast.

Nutrition: calories 179, fat 3.2, fiber 3.4, carbs 31.3, protein 6.5

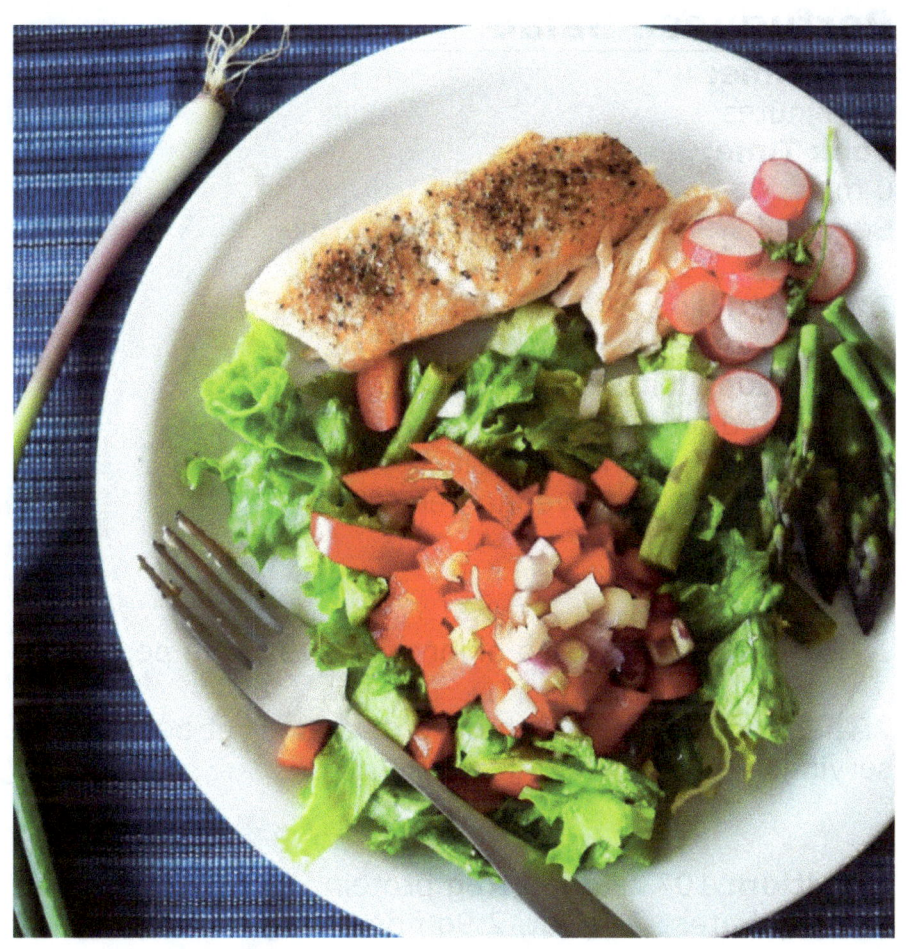

Portuguese Salad

Prep Time:
10 minutes
Cook Time:
0 min
Serve: 4

Ingredients:

- 3 cups tomatoes, sliced
- 2 red onions, peeled, sliced
- 2 tablespoons olive oil
- ½ teaspoon cayenne pepper

Directions:

1. Mix tomatoes with red onions, and cayenne pepper.

2. Then top the salad with olive oil and stir it before serving.

Nutrition: 107 calories, 1.8g protein, 10.5g carbohydrates, 7.4g fat, 2.9g fiber, 0mg cholesterol, 9mg sodium, 405mg potassium.

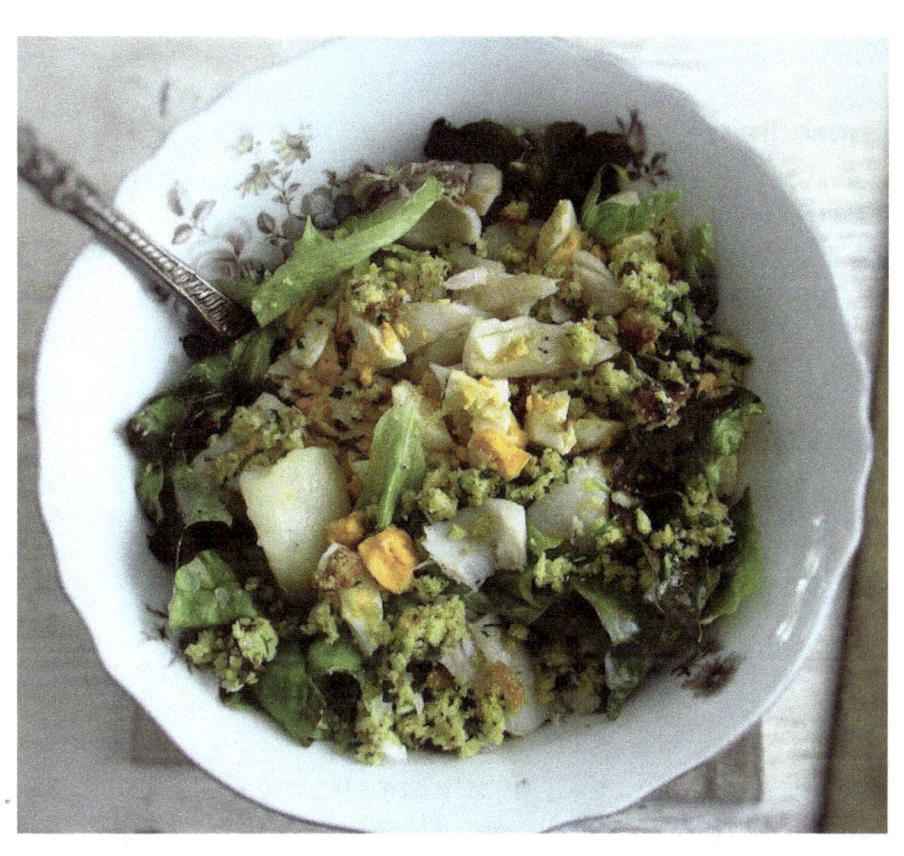

Tomato Eggs

Prep Time:
10 minutes
Cook Time:
15 minutes
Serve: 6

Ingredients:

- 12 eggs, beaten
- 2 cups tomatoes, chopped
- 2 tablespoons olive oil
- 1 teaspoon dried rosemary
- ½ teaspoon chili powder

Directions:

1. Preheat the olive oil in the skillet

2. Add tomatoes, dried rosemary, and chili powder.

3. Roast tomatoes for 10 minutes. Stir them from time to time.

4. After this, add eggs, gently stir the meal and cook it for 5 minutes more with the closed lid.

Nutrition: 178 calories, 11.6g protein, 29g carbohydrates, 3.3g fat, 13.6g fiber, 327mg cholesterol, 128mg sodium, 266mg potassium.

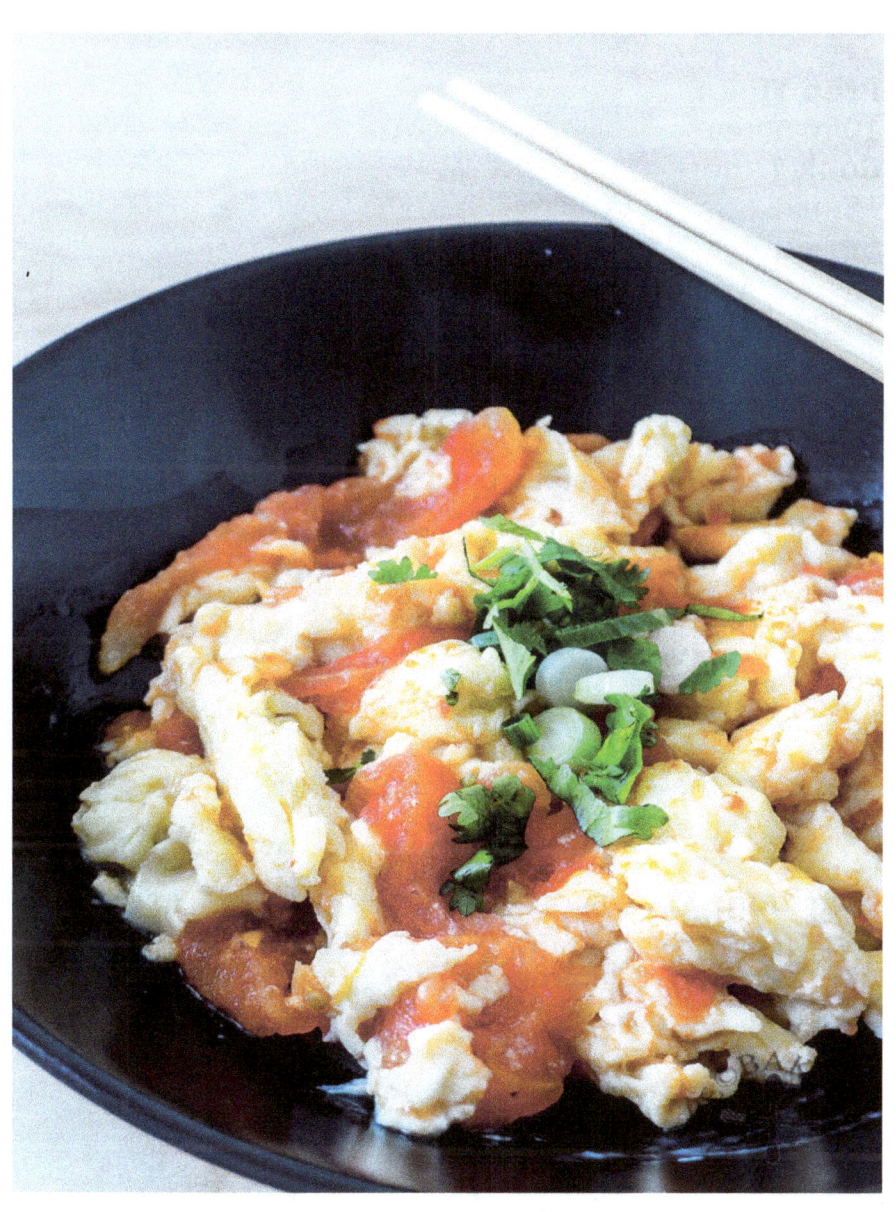

Vanilla Pears

Prep Time:
10 minutes
Cook Time:
15 min
Serve: 4

Ingredients:

- 2 cups of rice milk
- 4 pears, chopped
- 1 teaspoon vanilla extract

Directions:

1. Bring the rice milk to boil.

2. Add vanilla extract and chopped pears.

3. Simmer the meal for 5 minutes on medium heat.

Nutrition: 184 calories, 1g protein, 44.4g carbohydrates, 1.3g fat, 6.5g fiber, 0mg cholesterol, 45mg sodium, 278mg potassium.

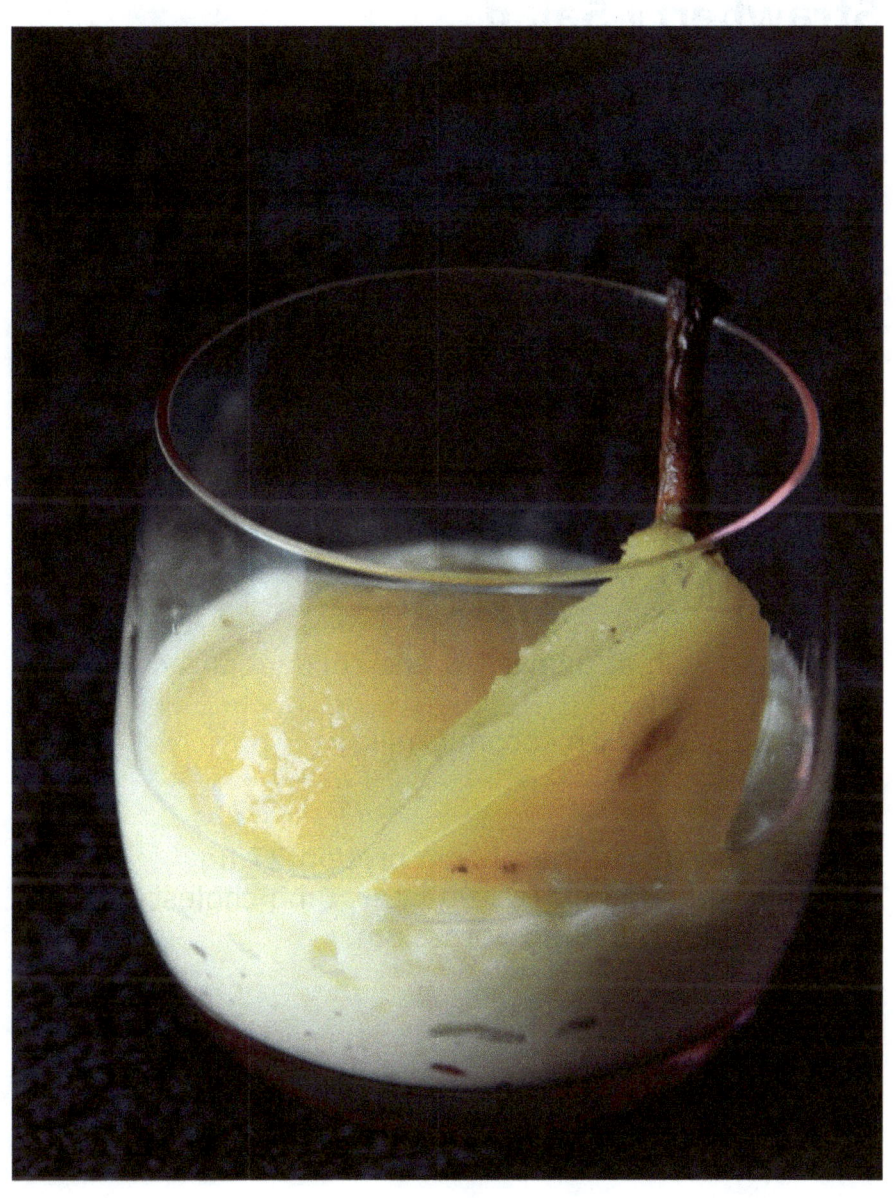

Strawberry Salad

Prep Time:
5 minutes
Cook Time:
0 minutes
Serve: 1

Ingredients:

- 2 oz nuts, chopped
- 1 cup strawberries, sliced
- 2 tablespoons coconut milk
- 1 teaspoon coconut shred

Directions:

1. Mix nuts with strawberries and coconut shred.

2. Top the salad with coconut milk.

Nutrition: 469 calories, 11.5g protein, 27.8g carbohydrates, 38.4g fat, 9g fiber, 0mg cholesterol, 386mg sodium, 638mg potassium.

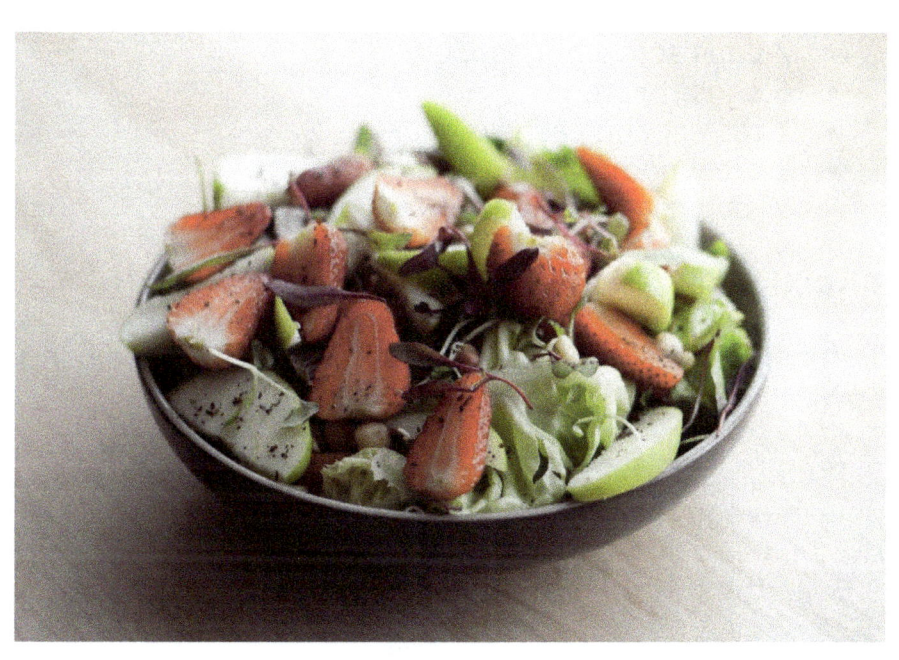

Spinach Frittata

Prep Time:
10 minutes
Cook Time:
30 minutes
Serve: 4

Ingredients:

- 2 cups spinach, chopped
- 6 eggs, beaten
- 1 tablespoon cashew butter
- 1 teaspoon chili powder
- ¼ cup coconut cream

Directions:

1. Mix all ingredients except cashew butter in the mixing bowl.

2. Then grease the baking pan with cashew butter and pour the egg mixture inside.

3. Bake the frittata at 350F for 30 minutes.

Nutrition: 158 calories, 9.9g protein, 29g carbohydrates, 3.3g fat, 12.3g fiber, 246mg cholesterol, 144mg sodium, 246mg potassium.

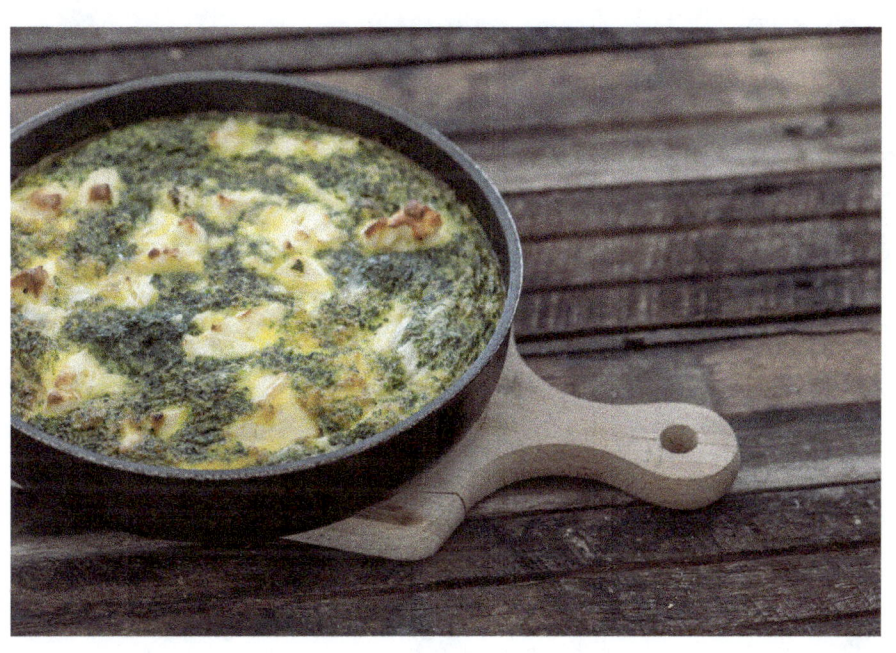

Granola Bars

Prep Time:
20 min
Cook Time:
0 min
Serve: 4

Ingredients:

- 7 oz pistachios, chopped
- 1 cup dates, pitted
- ½ cup raisins, chopped
- 2 tablespoons chia seeds

Directions:

1. Mix all ingredients in the bowl.

2. When the mixture is homogenous, transfer it in the baking paper and flatten it in the shape of a square.

3. Cut the granola into bars.

Nutrition: 479 calories, 12.7g protein, 64g carbohydrates, 25.6g fat, 11.6g fiber, 0mg cholesterol, 269mg sodium, 969mg potassium.

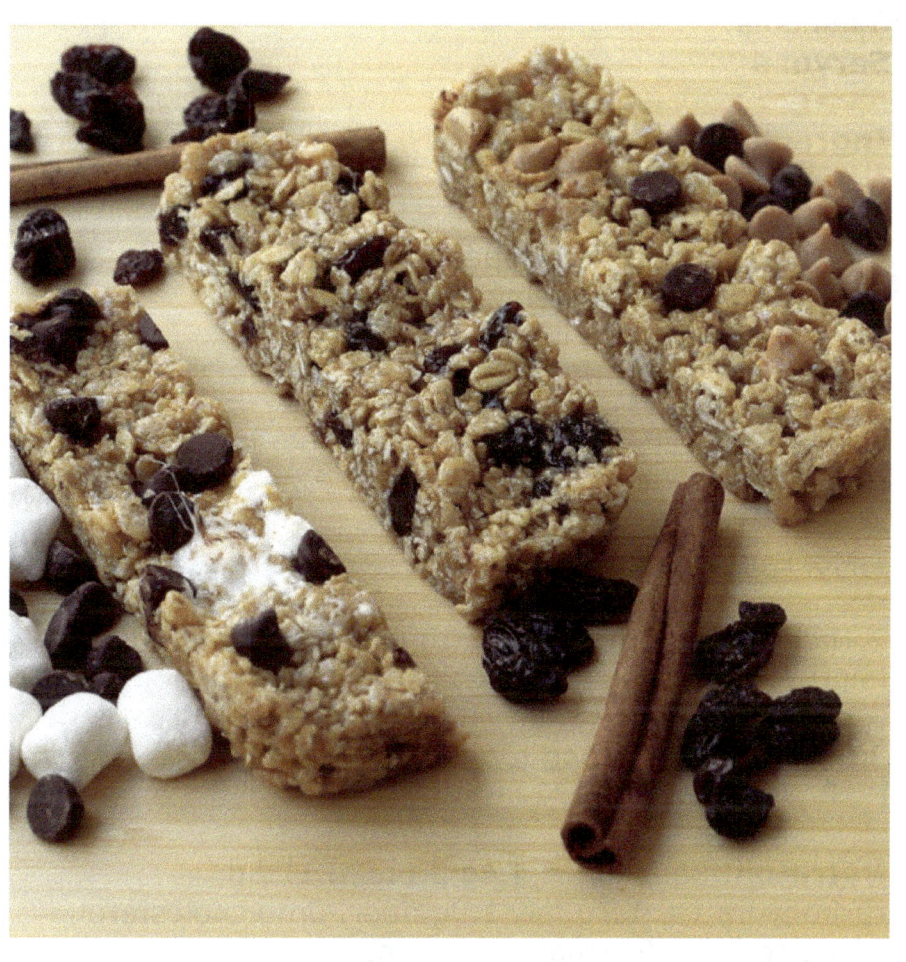

Kale Salad

Prep Time:
10 minutes
Cook Time:
0 minutes:
Serve: 4

Ingredients:

- 3 cups kale, chopped
- 2 cucumbers, chopped
- ¼ cup fresh parsley, chopped
- 2 tablespoons lemon juice
- ½ teaspoon dried mint
- 3 oz tofu, cubed

Directions:

1. Mix kale with cucumbers and parsley.

2. Then sprinkle the salad with lemon juice and dried mint.

3. Shake the salad and top it with tofu.

Nutrition: 66 calories, 4.4g protein, 11.5g carbohydrates, 1.2g fat, 1.9g fiber, 0mg cholesterol, 31mg sodium, 531mg potassium.

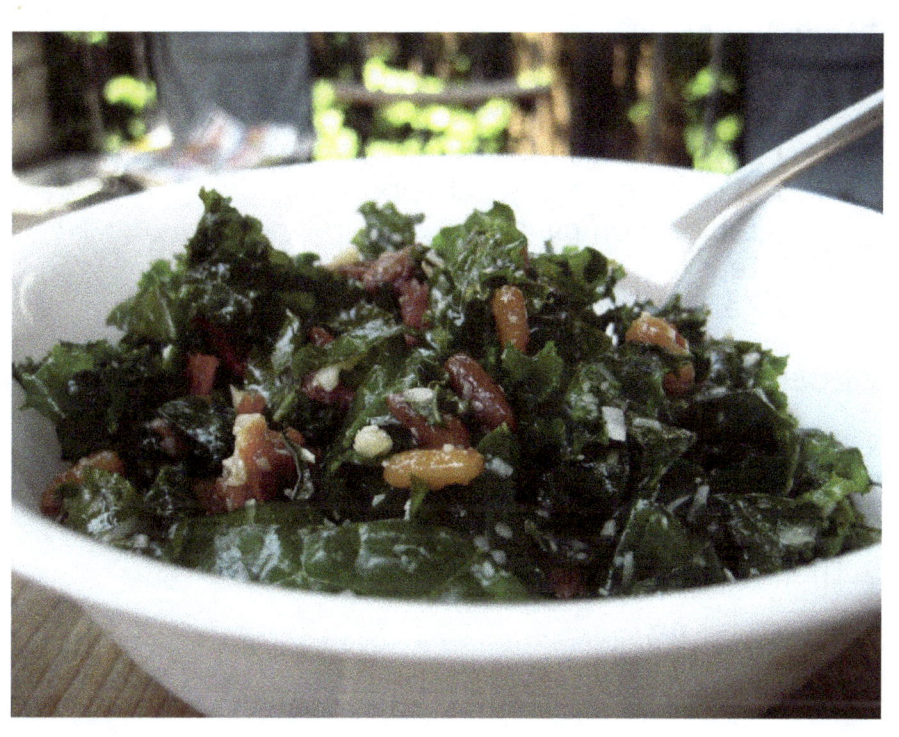

Quinoa Salad

Prep Time:
10 minutes
Cook Time:
0 minutes
Serve: 2

Ingredients:

- 2 cups quinoa, cooked
- 1 cup tomatoes, chopped
- 1 cup fresh parsley, chopped
- 1 tablespoon olive oil
- 1 teaspoon lemon juice
- 2 garlic cloves, diced

Directions:

1. In the salad bowl, mix quinoa with tomatoes, parsley, and garlic cloves.

2. Then add olive oil and lemon juice.

3. Stir the salad.

Nutrition: 718 calories, 25.9g protein, 115.5g carbohydrates, 17.8g fat, 14g fiber, 0mg cholesterol, 31mg sodium, 1352mg potassium.

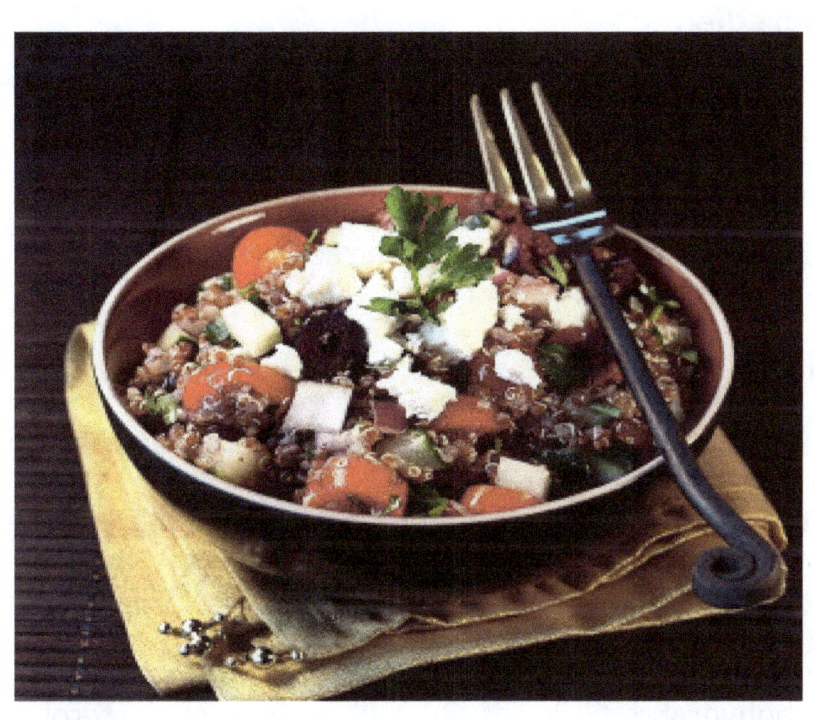

Shredded Carrot Bowl

Prep Time:
10 minutes
Cook Time:
0 minutes
Serve: 4

Ingredients:

- 3 cups carrot, shredded
- 3 oz raisins, chopped
- 3 tablespoons lemon juice
- 2 tablespoons olive oil
- 1 tablespoons dried cilantro
- 1 tablespoon raw honey

Directions:

1. Put all ingredients in the salad bowl and carefully mix.

2. Let the meal rest for at least 5 minutes before serving.

Nutrition: 176 calories, 1.5g protein, 29.9g carbohydrates, 7.2g fat, 2.9g fiber, 0mg cholesterol, 62mg sodium, 441mg potassium.

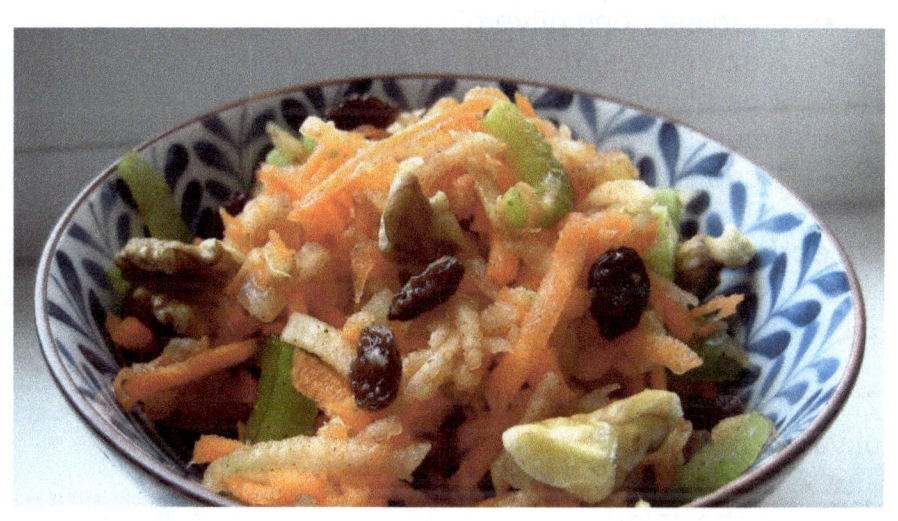

Italian Style Salad

Prep Time:
10 minutes
Cook Time:
0 minutes
Serve: 4

Ingredients:

- 1 tablespoon Italian seasonings
- 2 tablespoons olive oil
- 2 oz Parmesan, grated
- 2 oz olives, chopped
- 1 cup tomatoes, chopped
- 1 cup cucumbers, chopped

Directions:

1. Mix olives with tomatoes and cucumbers.

2. Then sprinkle the salad with Italian seasonings and olive oil.

3. Shake the salad.

4. Top it with parmesan.

Nutrition: 145 calories, 5.3g protein, 4.5g carbohydrates, 12.7g fat, 1.1g fiber, 13mg cholesterol, 259mg sodium, 148mg potassium.

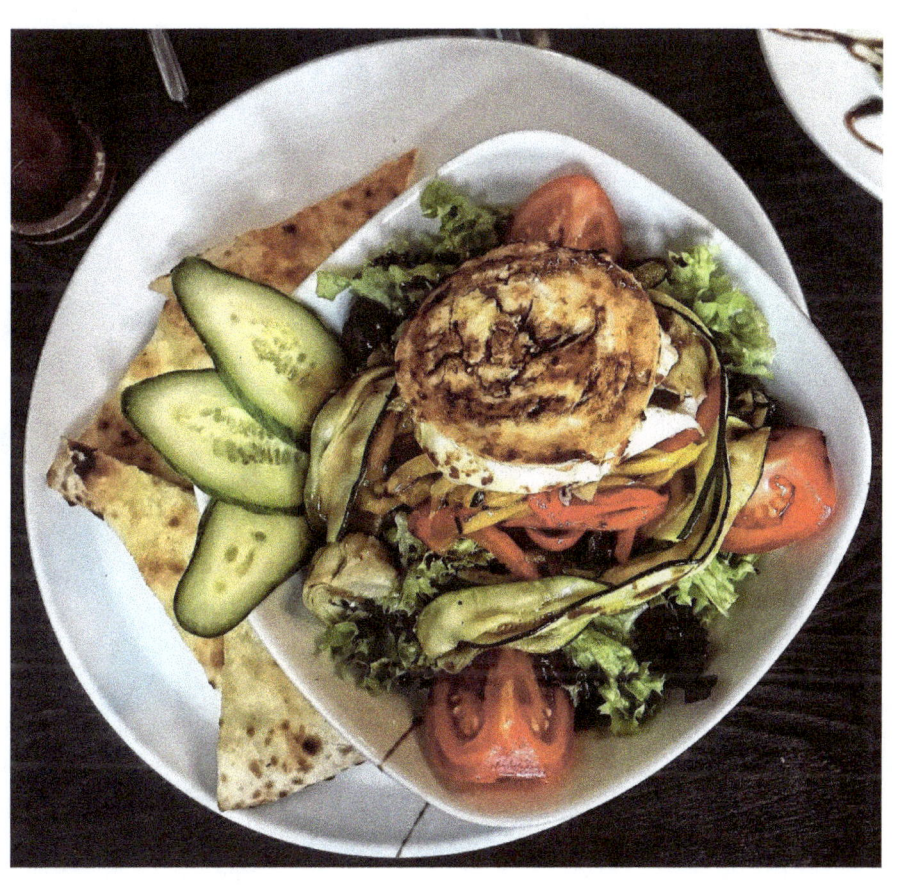

Sprouts Salad

Prep Time:
10 minutes
Cook Time:
0 minutes
Serve: 4

Ingredients:

- 1 red onion, sliced
- 2 cups bean sprouts
- 1 cup fresh cilantro, chopped
- 1 tablespoon lemon juice
- 1 teaspoon dried rosemary
- 1 tablespoon olive oil

Directions:

1. Put all ingredients in the salad bowl.

2. Shake the salad well.

Nutrition: 71 calories, 4.3g protein, 6.8g carbohydrates, 4.1g fat, 0.9g fiber, 0mg cholesterol, 9mg sodium, 241mg potassium.

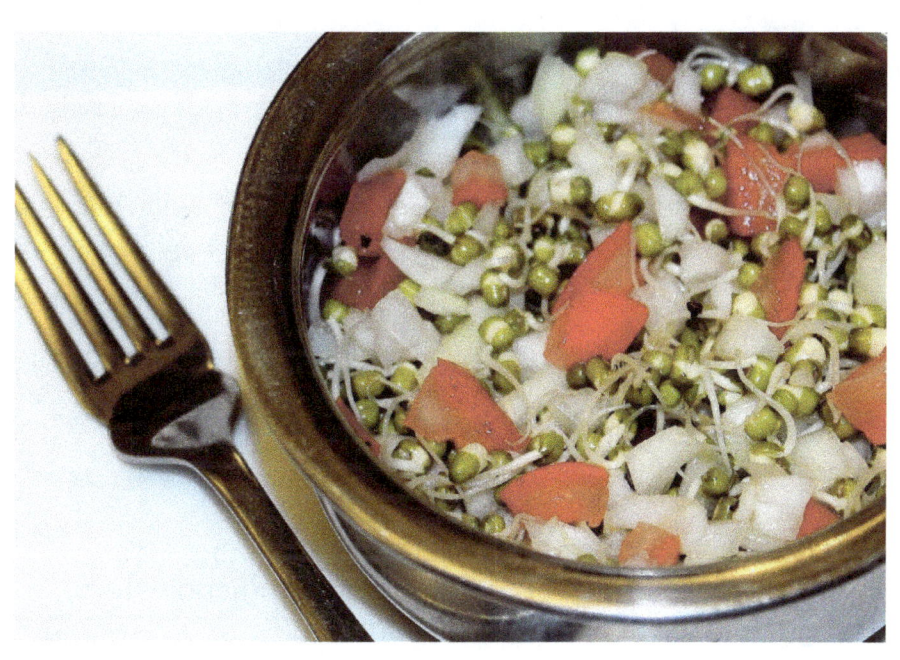

Corn Bowl

Prep Time:
10 minutes
Cook Time:
0 minutes
Serve: 4

Ingredients:

- 10 oz corn kernels, cooked
- 1 cup tomatoes, chopped
- 1 tablespoon fresh dill, chopped
- 1 tablespoon plain yogurt
- ½ cup radish, chopped

Directions:

1. Mix tomatoes with fresh dill, plain yogurt, and radish.

2. Then add corn kernels, gently stir the meal.

Nutrition: 345 calories, 13.4g protein, 75.5g carbohydrates, 4.7g fat, 11.4g fiber, 0mg cholesterol, 70mg sodium, 1215mg potassium.

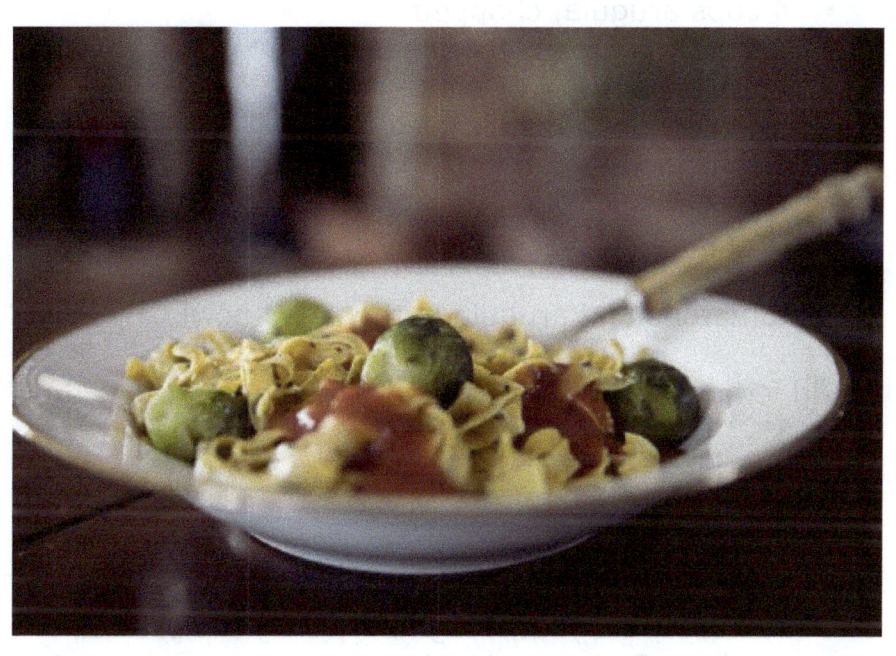

Lemon Tomatoes

Prep Time:
10 minutes
Cook Time:
0 minutes
Serve: 6

Ingredients:

- 4 cups arugula, chopped
- 4 cups tomatoes, chopped
- 2 tablespoons olive oil
- 3 tablespoons lemon juice
- 1 teaspoon lemon zest, grated

Directions:

1. Put tomatoes and arugula in the salad bowl.

2. Add lemon juice, olive oil, and lemon zest.

3. Stir the meal gently before serving.

Nutrition: 67 calories, 1.5g protein, 5.4g carbohydrates, 5.1g fat, 1.7g fiber, 0mg cholesterol, 11mg sodium, 344mg potassium.

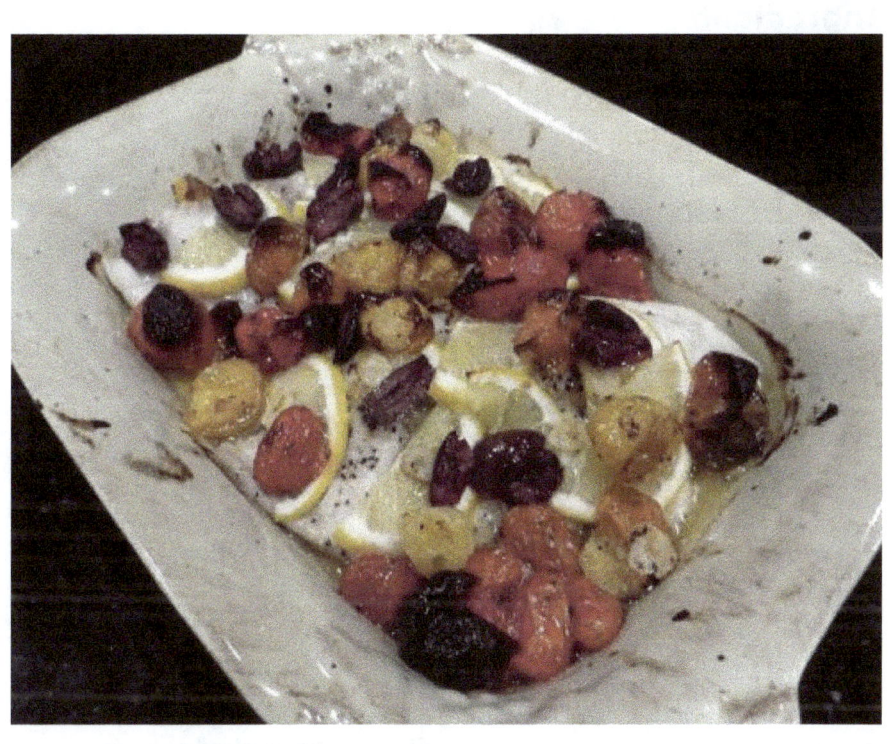

Avocado Salad

Prep Time:
10 minutes
Cook Time:
0 minutes
Serve: 4

Ingredients:

- 3 tomatoes, roughly chopped
- 2 avocados, pitted and chopped
- 1 cup parsley, chopped
- 1 teaspoon cayenne pepper
- ½ teaspoon dried rosemary
- 2 tablespoons olive oil

Directions:

1. In the salad bowl, mix tomatoes with avocados, parsley, and dried rosemary.

2. Then sprinkle the salad with olive oil and cayenne pepper. Gently shake the salad.

Nutrition: 289 calories, 3.2g protein, 13.5g carbohydrates, 27g fat, 8.5g fiber, 0mg cholesterol, 19mg sodium, 800mg potassium.

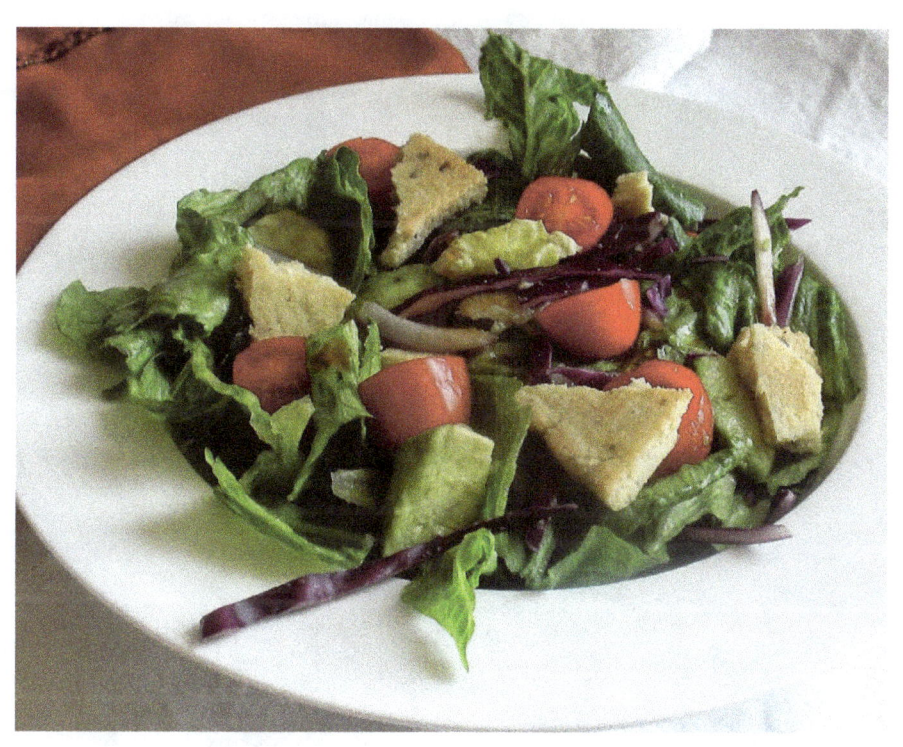

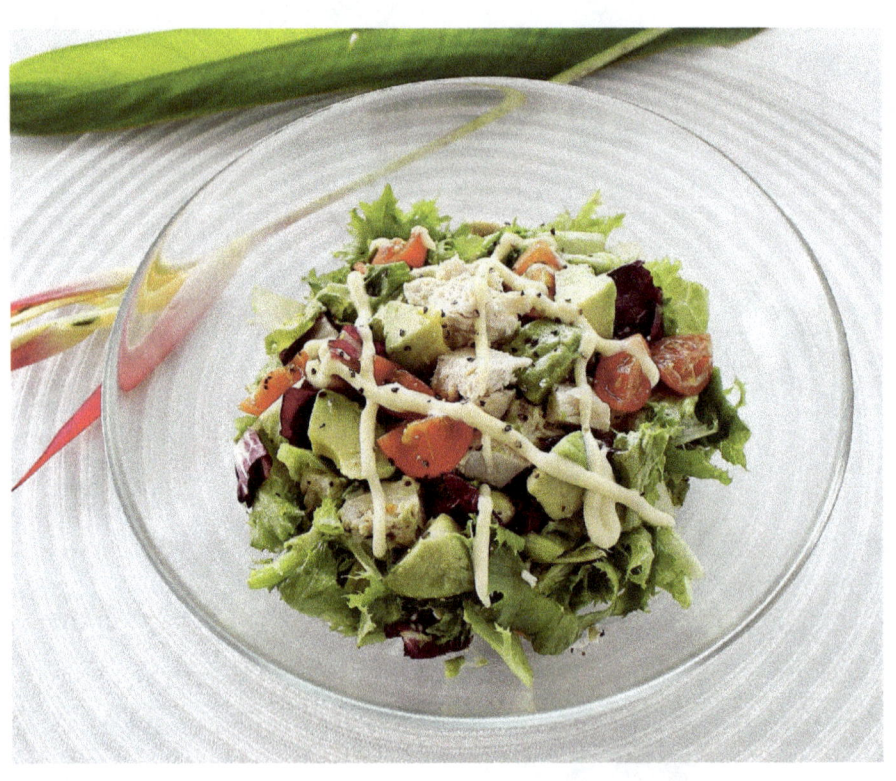

www.ingramcontent.com/pod-product-compliance
Lightning Source LLC
Chambersburg PA
CBHW070726030426
42336CB00013B/1926